Ouanassa Hamouda
Allaoua Hichem Fendri

Systemic candidiasis

Ouanassa Hamouda
Allaoua Hichem Fendri

Systemic candidiasis

ScienciaScripts

Imprint

Any brand names and product names mentioned in this book are subject to trademark, brand or patent protection and are trademarks or registered trademarks of their respective holders. The use of brand names, product names, common names, trade names, product descriptions etc. even without a particular marking in this work is in no way to be construed to mean that such names may be regarded as unrestricted in respect of trademark and brand protection legislation and could thus be used by anyone.

Cover image: www.ingimage.com

This book is a translation from the original published under ISBN 978-620-6-72532-9.

Publisher:
Sciencia Scripts
is a trademark of
Dodo Books Indian Ocean Ltd. and OmniScriptum S.R.L publishing group

120 High Road, East Finchley, London, N2 9ED, United Kingdom
Str. Armeneasca 28/1, office 1, Chisinau MD-2012, Republic of Moldova, Europe
Printed at: see last page
ISBN: 978-620-8-26327-0

Contents

INTRODUCTION - ISSUES

Invasive mycoses are opportunistic infections, responsible for significant morbidity and mortality among hospitalized patients (40%), which has led to a significant increase in the cost of hospital stays [1].

Among these invasive mycoses, systemic candidiasis comes to the fore, as its frequency is increasing to the benefit of other infections. *Candida spp* accounts for 70% to 90% of all invasive mycosis species [2]. It is the fourth most common cause of septicemia in the United States and the seventh most common cause in Europe [3,4]. Some *Candida* species are commensals of the human digestive tract and urogenital tract (*Candida albicans* and *Candida glabrata*), while others are saprophytes of the skin (*Candida parapsilosis*). Numerous other species of *Candida*, living as saprophytes in the external environment, can be found in humans in a commensal state on mucous membranes or the skin:

- *C. tropicalis*, a natural saprophyte (soil, water, cereals), is found in the digestive tract and urinary tract.

- *Candida famata* and *Candida guillermondii* are commensal skin yeasts.

- *C. krusei* and *Candida kefyr* (fermented dairy products) are food-borne species,

- *C. dublinensis* is found in AIDS patients.

The terminology used to describe this type of infection varies in the literature. Several terminologies have been used: deep-seated, systemic, invasive, visceral or disseminated candidiasis. Some authors have attempted to define systemic or invasive candidiasis as the presence of *Candida* yeast in a normally sterile site. Systemic candidiasis encompasses several clinical varieties: *Candida* septicemia (or candidemia), defined as infection proven by the presence of one or more *Candida-positive* blood cultures, and disseminated candidiasis, which corresponds to the presence of *Candida* in at least two non-contiguous organs or sites [5,6], most often secondary to hematogenous dissemination [7].

Systemic candidiasis occurs mainly in patients hospitalized in wards housing immunocompromised patients, i.e. intensive care units, onco-hematology units , transplant patients, burn patients and neonates.

Given their opportunistic nature, *Candida* only exerts its pathogenic power in the presence of favorable factors. There are three major pathogenic components in the development of systemic candidiasis:

- The increase in colonization resulting from the use of broad-spectrum antibiotics [2].
- Disruption of the normal skin barrier as a result of invasive equipment such as permanent intra-vascular catheters, recent surgery or trauma, severe mucositis associated with chemotherapy or cytotoxic radiotherapy.
- Immune dysfunction (e.g. neutropenia), which leads to diffusion and proliferation in deep tissue [8].

Candida spp can reach deep tissues in two ways: endogenously or exogenously.

Candida albicans remains the most frequently isolated species in these invasive infections. In recent years, however, the emergence of *non-albicans* species has been observed: *Candida glabrata, Candida parapsilosis Candida tropicalis, Candida krusei* and *Candida auris* have seen a marked increase in their frequency [9].

Systemic candidiasis remains a serious infection, despite advances in treatment. This is mainly due to the fact that diagnosis is often delayed and difficult to establish, given the polymorphous and non-specific symptomatology; it usually presents with fever of varying intensity, and may even lead to full-blown septic shock [10]. Only its persistence despite broad-spectrum antibiotic therapy can distinguish it from bacterial septicemia (if we exclude possible bacterial resistance to antibiotics). Only a positive *Candida* specimen from a sterile site, or histopathological evidence by tissue biopsy, can confirm the diagnosis of proven systemic candidiasis according to European Organization for Research and Treatment of Cancer (EORTC) criteria in immunocompromised patients [11].

Prognosis depends on the early administration of a specific, appropriate antifungal treatment.

To make the diagnosis of systemic candidiasis more sensitive and specific, new diagnostic methods have been developed, such as the determination of 1,3-ß-D-glucan and mannans, which are components of the *Candida* cell wall and can be detected in blood. The combined detection of mannan antigens and anti-mannan antibodies in blood can shorten the diagnostic delay compared with blood cultures, which lack sensitivity (around 50%) and are often positive at a late stage [11].

Molecular detection of *Candida* by PCR (polymerase chain reaction) could enable candidemia to be diagnosed with excellent sensitivity and specificity [12].

The prevalence of systemic candidiasis varies according to patient population. Despite increased awareness of this type of infection among clinicians, mortality remains high (40-60%). Epidemiological data from Algeria are not yet widely available. It is in this context that we felt it important to monitor the evolution of the epidemiology over time through a prospective descriptive study of all episodes of CS occurring at the CHU and CAC of BATNA between January 1er 2016 and December 31 2018 in order to improve medical practices both diagnostically and therapeutically.

The objectives of our study were:

Main objective

To describe the epidemiological characteristics of systemic *Candida* infections in high-risk wards at the University Hospital Center (CHU) and the Cancer Center.

(CAC) of BATNA.

Secondary objectives

- Identify and analyze risk factors for systemic candidiasis.
- Demonstrate the value of the colonization index in the occurrence of disseminated candidiasis.
- Describe the distribution of *Candida* species found.
- Estimate the mortality rate and the importance of therapeutic choice on disease progression.
- Describe the factors influencing the successful progression of the disease.
- Determine the value of the mannan antigen/anti-mannan antibody assay in differentiating between infection and colonization.
- Establish a well-coded management strategy for all deep-seated samples positive for *Candida spp*.

CANDIDA AND SYSTEMIC CANDIDIASIS: A REVIEW OF THE LITERATURE

1 CLASSIFICATION

1.1 Mushrooms-Definition

Fungi (fungi or mycetes) are cosmopolitan eukaryotic micro-organisms that can be single- or multi-cellular, including macroscopic (macromycetes) and microscopic (micromycetes) species, with a filamentous or yeast-like appearance [13].

Unlike the plant kingdom, fungi draw their energy from external organic matter, so they're heterotrophs. What's more, they lack chlorophyll, so they can't produce their own carbon by photosynthesis.

Mushrooms live in 3 main ways:

- Symbiosis: fungi live in mutually beneficial associations with other organisms.
- Parasitism: fungi grow on living organisms.
- Saprophytism: fungi take their nutrients from decomposing organic matter. They are very important as decomposers and recyclers of dead matter.

In the 1950s, around 70 parasitic fungi were known: 10 causing deep mycoses, 15 mucosal mycoses and 40-50 dermatophytes. By 2006, over 550 had been identified. This increase can be explained by the fact that they are opportunistic and that, with scientific progress, we are better able to identify them [14].

1.2 General characteristics

1.2.1 Morphological characteristics

The vegetative apparatus, or thallus, is made up of a tangle of very fine, branched filaments that together form a mycelium.

There are two types of filaments:

- Septate or septate filaments: called hyphae, they are regular in diameter (3 to 5µm), with septa formed at more or less regular intervals. Fungi with this type of thallus are called Septomycetes.
- Unpartitioned or siphoned filaments: of irregular diameter (5 to 15µm), characteristic of lower fungi or Siphomycetes.

In some cases, the thallus is reduced to a single cell: yeast.

Some fungi are dimorphic and tropical in distribution (e.g. Histoplasma capsulatum). They come in two forms:

- Saprophytic filamentous form in the environment, grows at 25°C.
- Forms yeast in the body in a parasitic state, grows at 37°C.

Black mushrooms contain melanin in sometimes high concentrations in the wall.

1.2.1.1 Nutrition

Fungi are aerobic, absorptive feeders, heterotrophs that draw their energy from pre-formed organic matter, which they use as a source of carbon and nitrogen. Some fungi require amino acids, mineral salts or vitamins (thiamine, biotin) for their development.

The pH for their growth is around 7.

1.2.2 Reproduction

Fungi reproduce by spores in two ways:

- Asexual reproduction (anamorphic): this is the most common and simplest form of reproduction, involving simple mitosis (binary division of the nucleus).
- Sexual reproduction (teleomorphic): involves the meeting of specialized filaments (plasmogamy), the conjugation of nuclei (karyogamy) and finally chromatic reduction (meiosis) followed by one or more mitoses.

The mode of reproduction, mainly sexual, is currently used to classify fungi (Taxonomy).

1.3 Classification of fungi [12]

The fungus takes its name from the isolated form in culture:

- The sexual or teleomorphic form
- The asexual or anamorphic form.
- When several aspects coexist in the asexual form, we speak of a synanamorph.
- When both sexual and asexual forms coexist, we speak of a holomorph.

In practice, it's the name of the sexed form that is used first in the classification of fungi. The mushroom kingdom is divided into divisions, which are in turn subdivided into classes. These include the orders that bring families together.

A family comprises genera that encompass species, which can be subdivided into varieties.

Names end in :

- Mycotina for divisions (Example: Ascomycotina).
- Fungi for classes (Example: Ascomycetes).
- The suffix - **ale** is used to designate orders (e.g. Saccharomycetales).
- The suffix - **aceae** for families (e.g. Saccharomycetaceae).
- The suffix - **adeae** for subfamilies.

Each mushroom has a name that follows the rules of binomial nomenclature (genus and species) laid down by Carl Von Linné in the 18ème century [12].

The Hawksworth, Sutton and Ainsworth (1970) classification, modified by Kwon Chung and Bennett (1992), then by de Hoog (1995), Alexopoulos, Mimms and Blackwell (1996), and Sutton, Fothergil and Rinaldi (1998) are the most widely used. (Fig. 1).

Four divisions are distinguished according to sexual reproduction: Mastigomycotina, Zygomycotina, Ascomycotina and Basidiomycotina. In addition, when sexual reproduction is unknown, the division is called Deuteromycotina or Fungi imperfecti.

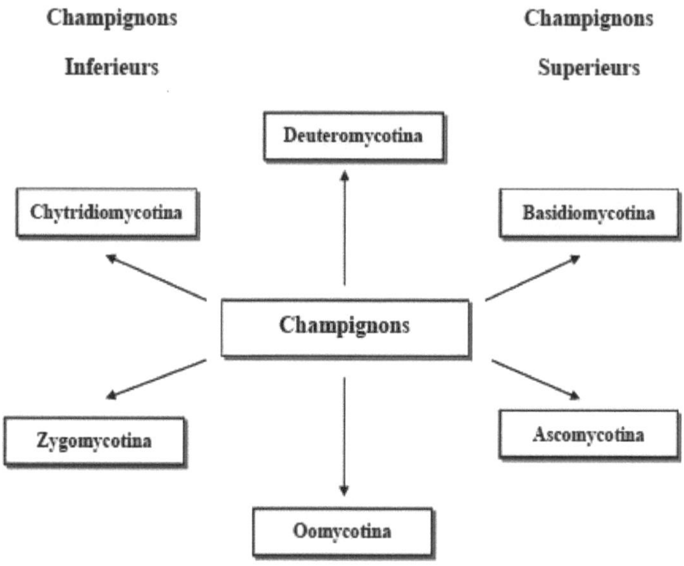

Figure. 1: General classification of fungi [12]

1.3.1 Mastigomycotina

- Very rarely involved in human pathology.
- Divided into two classes: Chytridiomycetes and Oomycetes.
- They are characterized by the presence of spores with flagella (one for Chytridiomycetes, two for Oomycetes) (Figure 2).
- Only the Chytridiomycetes will be included in the fungi kingdom, due to the presence of chitin in their walls and their nutrition, which is by absorption.

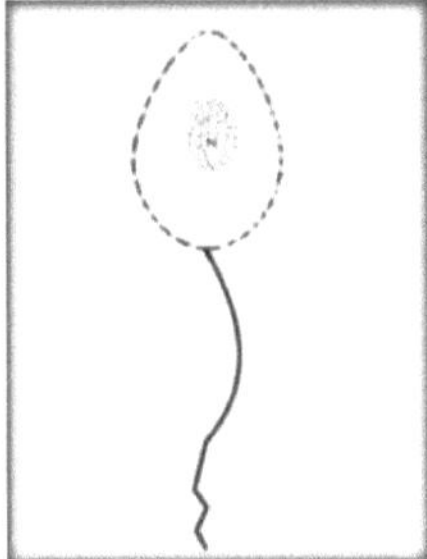

Figure. 2: Spore with flagellum of Chytridiomycetes [15].

1.3.2 The Zygomycotina

This division is characterized by the production of sexed spores called zygospores (Figure 3).

It includes numerous pathogens (Mucorales and Entomophthorales). Two characteristics distinguish them from the other so-called "higher" fungi (Ascomycotina and Basidiomycotina): the vegetative mycelium is larger, often dilated, with little or no partitioning, and asexual reproduction is said to be endogenous.

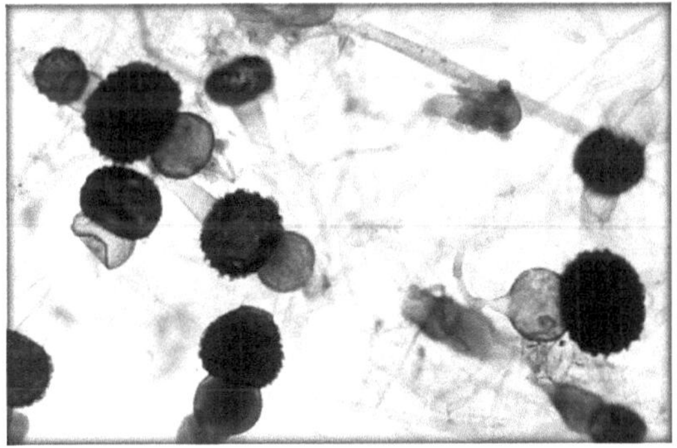

Figure. 3: Rhizopus zygospore [16]

1.3.3 The Ascomycotina

The spores resulting from sexual reproduction are called ascospores.

They are produced endogenously within a sac called the asca (Figure 4). They may be free-living (ascosporous yeasts or Hemiascomycetes) or produced inside a protective organ of variable shape called an ascocarp (true Ascomycetes or Euascomycetes).

11

This group includes a large number of human pathogens (Aspergillus, dermatophytes).

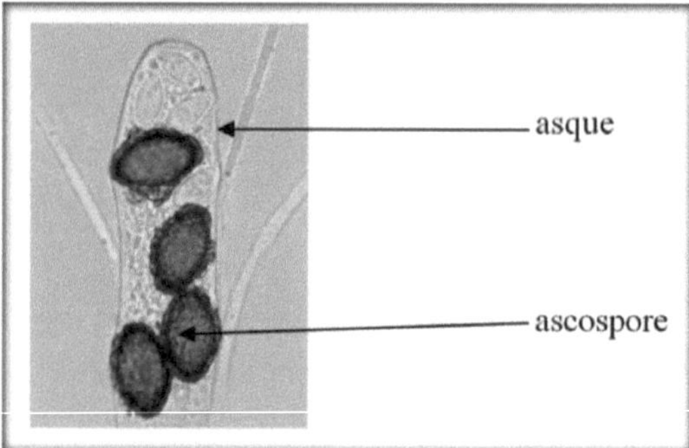

Figure. 4: Asque and Ascospore [17]

1.3.4 The Basidiomycotina

They are characterized by the production of sexualized spores called basidiospores, formed by the budding at the apex of elongated cells called basidia (Figure 5).

Basidiomycetes have a cloisonné thallus with "loops" in the partitions. The septa of the clamp-connected mycelial filaments usually include a single central pore with a complex structure known as a dolipore.

Basidiomycetes have little to do with human pathology; they are environmental saprophytes and sometimes plant pathogens.

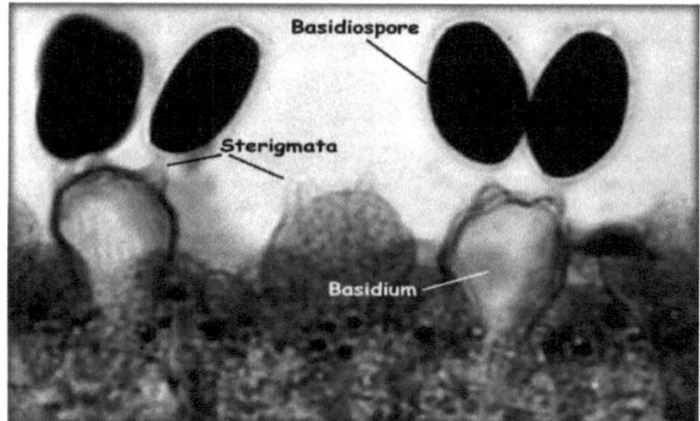

Figure. 5: Basidiospore and Basidium [18]

1.3.5 Deuteromycotina (imperfect fungi or Fungi imperfecti)

This division includes all species that multiply asexually.

The Deuteromycotina are divided into three classes (Figure 6):

- Blastomycetes: all yeast-like fungi.
- Hyphomycetes: all filamentous fungi with a septate thallus and free conidiogenous (spore- or conidium-producing) cells.
- Coelomycetes: filamentous fungi whose conidiogenous cells are contained in protective organs called pycnidia or acervuli.

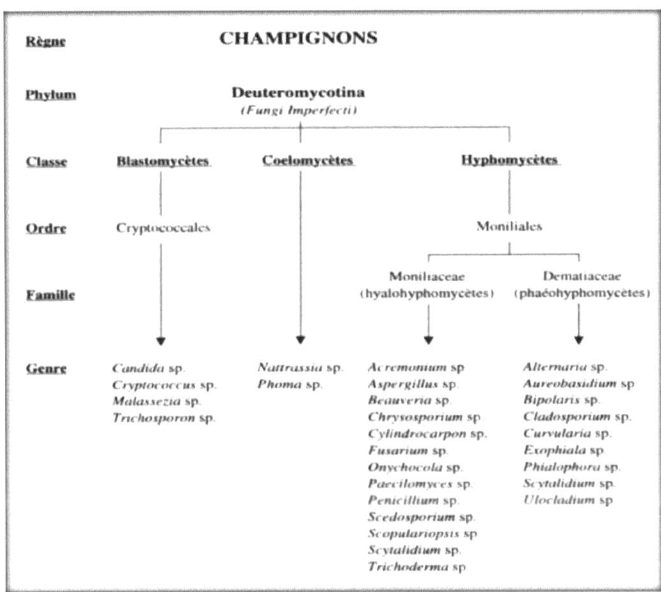

Figure. 6: Classification of the Deuteromycotina [19].

1.4 *Candida*'s place in the fungal kingdom

Today, the generally accepted classification of *Candida* is as follows [20] :

- Kingdom: Fungi.
- Division: Ascomycotina.
- Class: Ascomycetes.
- Sub&class: Hemiascomycetes.
- Order: Saccharomycetales.
- Family: Saccharomycetaceae.

- Genus: *Candida.*

Species of the genus *Candida* belong to two distinct groups:

- Species with a known sexual form, included in Ascomycetes, and whose sexual reproduction is by ascospores.
- Species with no known sexual form that are included in Deuteromycetes.

2 DESCRIPTION AND MORPHOLOGY OF *CANDIDA*

2.1 Main characteristics of *Candida*

2.1.1 Morphology

Candida are small, round or oval yeasts measuring 3-5µm, uncapped, unpigmented and aerobic.

They reproduce asexually by multilateral budding from the mother cell (the blastopore), forming smooth, shiny white or cream colonies (Figure 7).

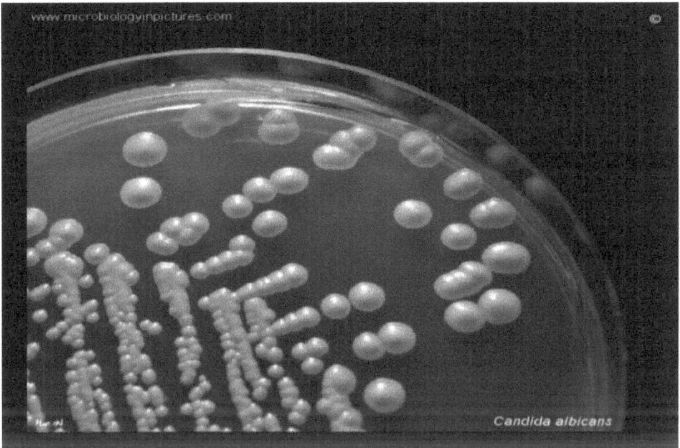

Figure 7: *Candida* morphology on Sabouraud medium [21].

Candida is polymorphic, and this polymorphism is influenced by the pH, temperature and richness of the culture medium, enabling it to evade the defenses associated with cellular immunity [13]. Thus, three morphological aspects can be encountered:

- The Blastospore form (Figure 8), round or oval, measuring from 2µm to 4 µm, sometimes with a forming bud.

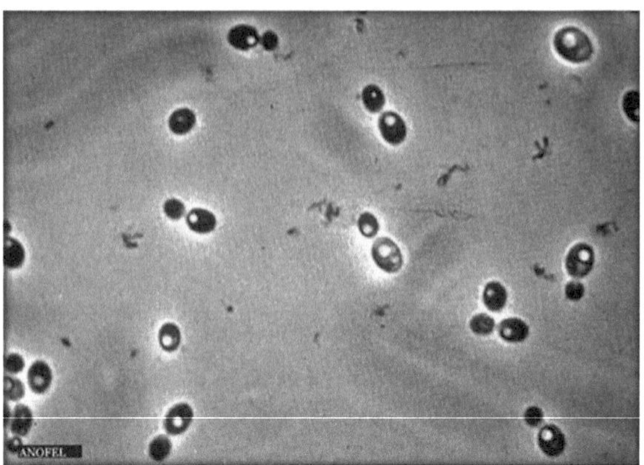

Figure 8: Blastospore of *Candida sp* p [22]

- The pseudomycelium form (Figure 9) : Composed of an assembly of cells measuring 500μm to 600μm, placed end to end to simulate a mycelial filament [14,23]. These cellular compartments are identical in length, and contain the same amount of genetic material, but differ in the amount of cytoplasm and these constituents [24].

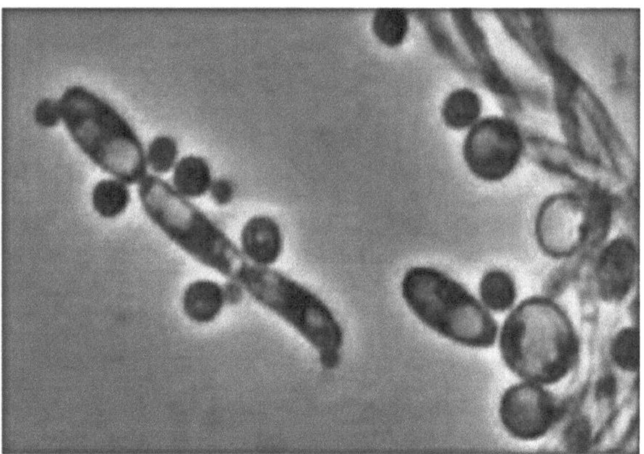

Figure 9: Pseudomycelium of *Candida albicans* [25]

- The true mycelium form (Figure 10): Specific to *the Candida albicans* species. The conversion of a yeast into a mycelial filament takes place via a structure called the germ tube. This form favors invasion of host tissues and organs [26].

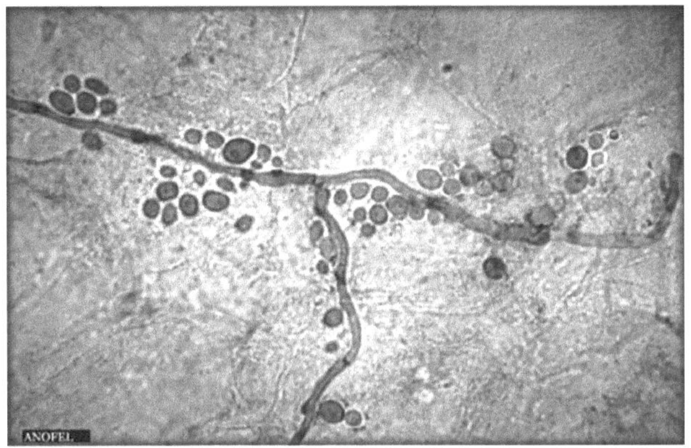

Figure. 10: Yeast and filaments (mycelium) [22]

- Chlamydospores (Figure 11) : These are rounded terminal or lateral structures formed by the thickening of the *Candida albicans* thallus under certain extreme environmental conditions of medium and temperature. They constitute a form of resistance and help to identify the organism , measure 10-15 µm and have a thick wall [27].

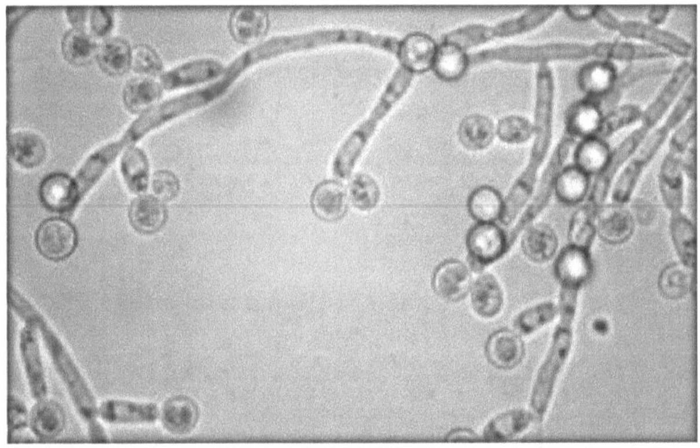

Figure. 11: Chlamydospores of *Candida albicans* [28]

2.1.2 *Candida* species and habitat

More than a dozen species of *Candida* are implicated in human pathology. The most common species remains *Candida albicans*, but in recent years we have seen the growing emergence of other opportunistic species, known as *"non-albicans"*.

The main pathogenic *Candida* species are :

2.1.2.1 *Candida albicans* [29]

- *Candida albicans* is the species most frequently incriminated in human pathology.
- It is an ovoid yeast with multilateral budding.
- It lives saprophytically in the digestive tracts of humans, mammals and birds.
- An opportunistic yeast, it becomes pathogenic under the influence of various factors.
- Dissemination is generally endogenous, originating in the digestive tract.

2.1.2.2 *Candida glabrata*

- It is a very small, round or ovoid yeast, measuring (2-3) x (3-4) μm.
- *Candida glabrata* is a saprophytic yeast of the human digestive and genitourinary tracts. In vaginal swabs, it takes second place to *Candida albicans*.
- *Candida glabrata* is a resistant opportunistic yeast, less sensitive to fluconazole and amphotericin B than most other *Candida* species. It has the ability and speed to develop resistance to all azoles [20].
- Its incidence is increased by sepsis in intensive care units.

2.1.2.3 *Candida parapsilosis*

- It is an ovoid-shaped yeast, measuring (3-4) x (3-7) μm.
- It is a saprophyte of the skin and can be responsible for cutaneous mycoses and onyxis.
- *Candida parapsilosis* has been implicated in septicemia caused by soiled catheters in patients with hematological malignancies [30].

2.1.2.4 *Candida tropicalis*

- Ovoid or globular yeast of variable size, measuring (4.5-7) x (6-10) µm.
- Saprophyte of the digestive and urinary tracts. It can also be found in the external environment: soil, water, cereals.
- It is the third most frequent yeast in the samples.
- In over 70% of cases, it is resistant to 5-fluorocytosine, but remains sensitive to azoles.
- *Candida tropicalis* is responsible for vaginitis and systemic candidiasis.

2.1.2.5 *Candida krusei*

- It is an elongated, ovoid or even cylindrical yeast, measuring (3-6) x (5-12) µm.
- It's a yeast found in dairy products and beer.
- The emergence of *C. krusei* is attributed to its primary resistance to fluconazole.
- This yeast is isolated in environments where fluconazole is used for prophylaxis.
- It is increasingly involved in pathological processes such as sepsis and visceral damage.
- Together with *Candida tropicalis*, it causes the classic triad of skin rash, fever and myalgia.

2.1.2.6 *Candida guilliermondii*

- It is an ovoid yeast, small in size, measuring (2-4) x (3-6) µm.
- It is isolated from air, seawater, food products and the digestive tracts of many animals and the urogenital tract of humans.
- It can cause skin mycoses such as plantar interdigital intertrigo and onyxis. It has been well documented to cause endocarditis in intravenous drug users and those undergoing surgical procedures, as well as fungemia in the immunocompromised.
- Neutropenia is the major risk of its emergence.

2.1.2.7 *Candida kefyr*

- It is an ovoid or elongated yeast measuring (3-5) x (7-10) μm.
- It is a saprophyte of human skin and respiratory mucosa. It is isolated from fermented dairy products.
- It can cause abscess-like lung infections and septicemia.

2.1.2.8 **Candida lusitaniae**

- This is a new opportunistic yeast, ovoid in shape and measuring (2-6) x (3-10) μm.
- It is mainly isolated from the digestive tracts of many animals, including pigs, warthogs and birds.
- It is often the most important cause of fungemia in patients with hematological malignancies. It is mentioned in the literature as a yeast capable of developing resistance to amphotericin B. The vital prognosis of this yeast is linked to the underlying terrain and its primary resistance to amphotericin B.

2.1.2.9 *Candida dubliniensis* [30]

- This is a new species of *Candida*, identified in 1995.
- Morphologies similar to those of *Candida albicans*, causing significant problems for identification.
- The majority of *Candida dubliniensis* isolates have been found in the oral cavity of HIV-infected subjects. However, this species has recently been isolated from other sites including the lung, vagina and blood of both HIV-infected and HIV-uninfected subjects.

2.1.2.10 *Candida norvegensis*

- Yeast isolated in Norway, hence its name.
- Uncommon in the outdoor environment, it has mainly been isolated from pulmonary and digestive samples.
- It's a yeast that's more likely to be found in hospital departments.
- Four cases of candidemia have been reported in the literature, all of them resistant to fluconazole.

2.1.2.11 *Candida famata*

- This yeast is widespread in the external environment and isolated mainly in humans from the skin.
- It is responsible for onyxis and plantar interdigital intertrigos.
- This yeast has also been implicated in central line-associated sepsis in bone marrow transplant patients.

2.1.2.12 *Candida auris*

- This yeast was first identified in 2009 from a strain isolated from the outer ear of a Japanese patient.
- *Candida auris* is capable of causing severe, invasive candidiasis by infecting the bloodstream, central nervous system and various internal organs.
- Its treatment is complicated by the fact that it is difficult to identify and easily confused with *Candida haemulonii*, *Candida famata* and others. What's more, *C. auris* is often multi-resistant to common antifungal agents.

2.1.2.13 *Candida africana*

Candida africana was initially described as an atypical Chlamydospore-negative variant of *C. albicans* [31], but was proposed as a new species on the basis of morphological, biochemical and physiological differences [32,33].

While subsequent molecular analyses have supported a varietal distinction (*C. albicans var. Africana*) [34]. The taxonomic status of *C. africana* remains controversial.

The *C. africana* isolates studied to date would have grown and produced hyphae more slowly than *C. albicans* or *C. dubliniensis* and could be distinguished from both by an inability to assimilate several sugars or to produce Chlamydospores and by appearance on chromogenic agars [31,32].

Moreover, despite an almost worldwide distribution, the overwhelming majority of *C. africana* isolates have been recovered from female genital samples [35].

Epidemiological analyses of *C. africana* have been hampered by the failure of commercially available identification methods to distinguish it from *C. albicans*. However, studies using PCR amplicon length analysis of the

Hwp-1 gene revealed that *C. africana* constituted 7.2% of complex *C. albicans* isolates from three different hospitals in southern Italy, a prevalence 3 times higher than that of *C. dubliniensis* in samples mainly from non-sterile sites from the same cohort of hospitalized patients [36].

2.1.3 Cellular and molecular organization

2.1.3.1 Intracellular structure

Candida are eukaryotic yeasts with all the following intracellular organelles:

- A nucleus, bounded by a double nuclear membrane, and containing eight chromosomes [37].
- A nucleolus.
- An endoplasmic reticulum.
- Golgi apparatus.

The vaculo - vesicular system is the only structure differentiating yeast from a classical eukaryotic cell, in relation to the cell cycle and division [24], and involved for the most part in wall synthesis [38].

2.1.3.2 The wall

The yeast wall (Figure 12) is a complex stratified structure [39]. Yet this structure is constantly evolving: a minor change in pH, temperature, salt or amino acid in the surrounding environment generates modifications in several hundred transcripts involved in wall biogenesis, leading to radical changes in shape and, a fortiori, in the molecules expressed [40].

The cell wall (the outermost part of the cell) is an impermeable membrane that maintains the yeast's morphological characteristics, and enables the yeast's first physical interactions with its environment.

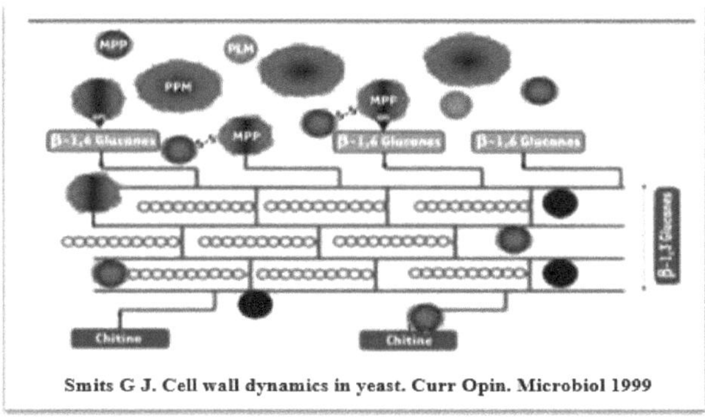

Figure. 12: Schematic representation of the *Candida albicans* wall [41].

- Glucans:

These are major constituents of the cell wall, accounting for 47% to 60% of its dry weight. It is a rigid microfibrillar skeleton made up of β-1,3 glucans forming a three-dimensional network attached to chitin by glycosidic bonds with lateral branches of β-1,6 glucans [42]. Glucans can be secreted into the blood of infected patients, where they exert toxicity up to and including anaphylactic shock in mice. In addition, *Candida albicans* glucans can directly inhibit monocyte function and indirectly inhibit T-cell function, suggesting their predominant role in the development of candidiasis [43].

- Mannoproteins (MPP):

They are linked to the microfibrillar backbone by non-covalent bonds such as phosphopeptidomannan (PPM), or by covalent bonds enabling their association either to other parietal proteins via disulfide (S-S) bridges, or to β-1,6 glucans via a partial GPI anchor or, as in the case of PIR proteins (proteins with internal repeats), directly to β-1,3 glucans. These different mannoproteins feature α-Man (red) and β-Man (green) epitopes (Figure12). Together with glucans, they are the major constituents of the wall, accounting for around 40% of polysaccharides and are the main participants in the formation of the wall matrix [42,44].

In humans, mannans and glucans elicit antibodies to varying degrees in healthy subjects, colonized or infected patients [45,46]. In this way, they confer antigenic properties on the cell wall that can alert the host's immune system.

- Phospholipomannan (PLM):

Surface glycolipid, possesses only β-Man epitopes (green) (Figure. 12). Phopholipomannans are interesting lipids, interacting with specific antibodies directed against oligommanosides [47]. Phopholipomannans are glucosamine-deficient, and possess their own glucan chain organization [48]. It has also been suggested that these compounds are involved in adhesion, protection and signalling mechanisms in *Candida albicans*.

- Chitin:

Along with glucans, it contributes to the composition of the wall skeleton and is involved in wall rigidity. In yeast, it is involved in the budding process and, in particular, in the formation of the constriction ring that separates the mother cell from the daughter cell [49]. Chitin is also involved in the formation of mycelial septa. Despite its major role, it is a minor wall constituent (0.6% to 9%) [50].

- Phosphopeptidomannan (PPM):

More commonly known as mannan, it is non-covalently associated with the wall surface. This high polymer of mannose (D-mannopyranose) is the quantitatively and qualitatively major yeast antigen [51]. Mannose residues are attached to a protein chain either by N-glycosidic linkage to an asparagine, or by O-glycosidic linkage to a serine or threonine.

2.2 Phathogenic mechanisms and virulence factors

2.2.1 Pathogenicity

The pathogenicity of *Candida* yeast is linked to a wide range of virulence factors and physical conditions (Figure 13). Virulence factors involved in *Candida* phathogenicity include morphological transition between yeast and hyphal forms, expression of adhesins and invasins on the cell surface, thigmotropism, biofilm formation and secretion of hydrolytic enzymes. In addition, fitness attributes include rapid adaptation to environmental pH fluctuations, metabolic flexibility, powerful nutrient acquisition systems and robust stress response mechanisms [50].

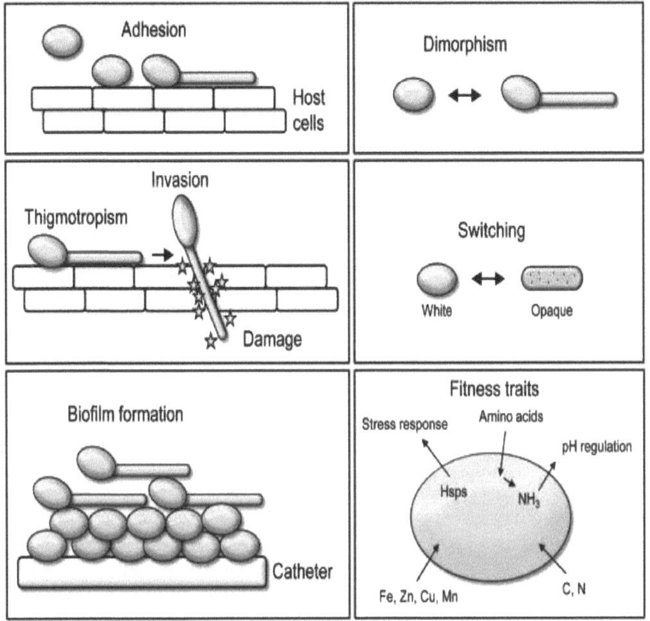

Figure. 13: Overview of the mechanisms of *Candida albicans* phathogenicity [50].

2.2.1.1 Polymorphism

Candida albicans is a fungus that can develop in several forms [52].

We distinguish :

- The ovoid budding yeast form.
- Elongated ellipsoidal cells with constrictions at the septa (pseudohyphae).
- True hyphae with parallel walls.
- Other morphologies include opaque white cells and Chlamydospores, which are thick-walled spore-like structures [53].

Yeast and hyphal forms are regularly observed during infection and have distinct functions, the role of pseudohyphae and in vivo switching is rather unclear and Chlamydospores have not been observed in patient samples [23,54].

Several environmental conditions can affect the morphology *of C. albicans*; citing for example:

- Changes in pH: at low pH (<6), *C. albicans* cells grow predominantly in yeast form, while at high pH (>7), hyphal growth is induced [55].
- In addition, the presence of N-acetylglucosamine, physiological temperature and CO_2 promote hyphal formation [56].

Candida albicans morphogenesis is regulated by Quorum Sensing (QS), a cell density-dependent fungal communication mechanism involved in the regulation of several fungal behaviors, such as virulence factor secretion and biofilm formation.

This fungal QS system was revealed ten years ago after the discovery of farnesol, which controls *Candida albicans* filamentation and plays multiple roles in its physiology as a signaling molecule and inducing adverse effects on host cells and other microbes. In addition to farnesol, aromatic alcohol-tyrosol is also a *Candida albicans* QS molecule controlling growth, morphogenesis and biofilm formation [57,58].

The transition between yeast and hyphal growth forms is known as dimorphism, and it has been proposed that both growth forms are important for phathogenicity [58]. The hyphal form has been shown to be more invasive than the yeast form [52], and represents the form mainly involved in diffusion [59].

2.2.1.2 Adhesins and invasins

Adhesion of *Candida albicans* cells to other microorganisms, abiotic surfaces and host cells is mediated by a specialized set of proteins (adhesins) [60,61].

The best-studied adhesins are the agglutinin-like sequence (ALs), a family of eight proteins (Als1-7 and Als9). The ALs genes encode cell-surface glycoproteins linked to glycosyl phosphatidyl inositol (GPI). Of the eight Als proteins, the hyphae-associated adhesin Als3 is particularly important for adhesion [62,63].

Hwp1 is another *Candida albicans* adhesin, associated with hyphae-associated GPI [62, 64,65].

Hwp1 and Als3 have also been shown to contribute to biofilm formation by acting as complementary adhesins [66].

Other proteins that do not influence morphology may also contribute to adhesion:

- GPI-associated proteins (Eap1, Iff4 and Ecm33).
- Wall-associated proteins (Mp65, putative β-glucanase, Phr1, β-1,3 glucanosyltransferase).
- Proteases associated with the cell surface (Sap9, Sap10).
- The integrin-type surface protein Int1 [67,68].

Candida albicans can use two mechanisms to invade the host cell. These are: induced endocytosis and active penetration [67, 68, 69,70]. For induced endocytosis, the fungus expresses specialized cell-surface proteins (invasins) that interact with E-cadherin on epithelial cells [63], and N-cadherin on endothelial cells, triggering engulfment of the fungal cell in the host cell. Indeed, even killed hyphae are taken up, indicating that induced endocytosis is a passive process that does not require viable fungal cells [70,71].

Two invasins have been identified to date, Als3 and Ssa1 [71,72]. Active penetration, on the other hand, requires viable hyphae of *Candida albicans* [70,73]. Secreted aspartic proteases (Saps) have also been proposed to contribute to active penetration.

2.2.1.3 Biofilm formation

Biofilm formation is another virulence factor for *Candida albicans*. Biofilm can form either on abiotic surfaces such as catheters and dentures, or on biotic surfaces such as mucous membranes [74].

Biofilms are formed in a sequential process including the adhesion of yeast cells to the substrate, the proliferation of these yeast cells, the formation of hyphae in the upper part of this biofilm, the accumulation of extracellular matrix and finally the dispersion of the yeast cells from the biofilm complex [63].

Mature biofilms are much more resistant to antimicrobial agents and host immune factors [74,75].

Dispersal of yeast cells from mature biofilms has been shown to contribute directly to virulence. The major heat shock protein Hsp90 was recently identified as a key regulator of dispersal in *Candida albicans* biofilms [76]. In addition, Hsp90 was also required for resistance to biofilm antifungals [76].

Several transcription factors control biofilm formation. These factors are : Bcr1, Tec1 and Efg1 [77]. In a recent study, Nobile et al, investigated the transcriptional network regulating biofilm formation and identified other previously unknown regulators of biofilm production [67]. These new factors include Ndt80, Rob1 and Brg1. Deletion of any of these regulatory factors results in defective biofilm formation [67].

2.2.1.4 Contact detection and thigmotropism

Thigmotropism is the contact detection that triggers hyphae and biofilm formation in *Candida albicans*. Upon contact with a surface, yeast cells switch to hyphal growth [77]. On certain substrates, such as agar or mucous surfaces, these hyphae can then invade the substrate. Contact with solid surfaces induces biofilm formation [75]. On surfaces with particular topologies (such as ridges), directional hyphal growth can be observed [78].

Brand et al demonstrated that the thigmotropism of *Candida albicans* hyphae is regulated by the uptake of extracellular calcium by calcium channels [79].

2.2.1.5 Hydrolase secretion

Following adhesion to host cell surfaces and hyphal growth, hyphae secrete hydrolases, which facilitate active penetration into these cells [79]. In addition, secreted hydrolases increase the efficiency of extracellular nutrient acquisition [80]. The classes of hydrolases secreted by *Candida albicans* are: proteases, phospholipases and lipases.

2.2.1.6 Adaptation to pH change

In the human body, *Candida albicans* is exposed to a surrounding pH ranging from slightly alkaline to acidic [81]. This pH change can cause severe stress to *Candida albicans*, including dysfunction of pH-sensitive proteins and impaired nutrient acquisition [81]. Among the first proteins identified as important for adaptation to pH change were the two cell wall β-glycosidases Phr1 and Phr2 [81] Phr1 is expressed at neutral-alkaline pH. In contrast, Phr2 is predominantly expressed at acidic pH [82].

Candida albicans is not only able to sense and adapt to environmental pH, but can also modulate extracellular pH, actively alkalinizing its surrounding environment to acquire nutrients and thus self-induce hyphal formation [83,84].

The underlying molecular mechanisms seem to involve the uptake of amino acids and probably other amine-containing molecules, such as polyamines, in the absence of glucose. *Candida albicans* then cleaves these substrates intra-cellularly with urea amidolyase, which induces alkalinization of the extracellular medium, and consequently hyphal morphogenesis [83].

Hyphae formation is considered a key virulence factor for *Candida albicans*, as non-filamentous mutants are less virulent. All these features contribute to its remarkable ability to coexist as a commensal and prevail as a fungal pathogen in humans.

2.2.1.7 Metabolic adaptation

Nutrition is an essential and fundamental condition for the survival and growth of all living organisms. Glycolysis, gluconeogenesis and responses to starvation are thought to contribute to host colonization and pathogenesis. In healthy individuals, *Candida albicans* is mainly found in the gastrointestinal microbiome. Although the concentration of nutrients in this environment may be naturally high, it is believed that the growth of the fungus is controlled by competition with the intestinal microbial flora.

During disseminated candidiasis in susceptible subjects, *Candida albicans* gains access to the bloodstream. Blood is relatively rich in glucose, the preferred nutrient source for most fungi [85]. However, phagocytic cells (macrophages and neutrophils) can effectively phagocytose *Candida albicans*.

Once inside a macrophage or neutrophil, the nutritional environment changes completely for the fungus. Not only do phagocytes produce highly reactive intermediates such as ROS, reactive nitrogen species (RNS) and antimicrobial peptides (AMP), but they also restrict nutrient availability, creating an environment of nutrient starvation [86].

For the adaptation of *Candida albicans* to a hostile host environment within macrophages, the fungus first switches from glycolysis to gluconeogenesis. Lipids and amino acids are proposed as nutrient sources in macrophages [87]. The fungus develops means of escape from macrophages by inhibiting the production of antimicrobial effectors and inducing hyphal formation. Hyphae formed inside phagocytic cells can penetrate the host immune cell by mechanical forces, enabling escape [87,88].

During systemic candidiasis, fungal cells can spread to virtually any organ in the human host. In the liver, for example, *Candida albicans* has access to large quantities of glycogen (the main glucose storage molecule). In other tissues, *Candida albicans* is confronted with relatively low glucose concentrations and uses alternative metabolic pathways to utilize host proteins, amino acids, lipids and phospholipids. The fungus can use secreted proteases to hydrolyze host proteins.

In summary, during infection, the main sources of nutrients for *Candida albicans* are probably host-derived glucose, lipids, proteins and amino acids, depending on the anatomical niche. In order to utilize these different nutrients, *Candida albicans* has the ability to respond rapidly and dynamically to host-induced changes, which contributes to its success as a pathogen [89].

3 RISK FACTORS FOR CANDIDA INFECTIONS

The development of severe *Candida* infection requires the intervention of several risk factors. Among these factors, however, some are more specific and merit particular attention [90, 91, 92,93].

These risk factors are divided into two sub-groups: major risk factors and minor risk factors. (Table I).

Table. I: Risk factors predisposing to the development of systemic candidiasis

Major risk factors	Minor risk factors
<ul><li>Colonization of several body sites</li><li>Broad-spectrum antibiotics</li><li>Immunossupression</li><li>Vascular approaches</li><li>Extensive burns (> 50%)</li><li>Major surgery</li><li>Digestive perforation</li><li>Hemodialysis</li><li>Major trauma</li><li>Neutropenia</li></ul>	<ul><li>Extreme age (prematurity and old age).</li><li>Diabetes</li><li>Renal insufficiency</li><li>Recent surgery</li><li>Bladder probe</li><li>Stay in intensive care> 7 days</li><li>Candidiasis >10^5 UFC /ml</li></ul>

[Eggimann P, et al. Candidoses en réanimation Réanimation .2002 ; 11 : 209-21© 2002 Éditions scientifiques et médicales Elsevier SAS]

3.1 Major risk factors
3.1.1 Colonization

Colonization with yeasts of the *Candida* genus is considered a very important risk factor [94].

In the early 1980s, Solomkin et al's work on peritonitis in non-neutropenic patients showed that the number of colonized body sites is proportional to the risk of developing an invasive infection. It was on this basis that the prescription of empirical treatment was recommended as soon as the number of colonized sites exceeded two [95].

According to epidemiological data, the proportion of colonized patients increases after 7 days, reaching 50% to 70%. Only 1% to 5% will develop an invasive infection [96,97].

Obviously, the discovery of colonization alone is not sufficient to initiate antifungal therapy. In surgical resuscitation, the degree of colonization and an Apache II score above 20 were independently predictive of the development of severe infection [98].

Eggimann and Pittet carried out a study of candidiasis in intensive care units, and found that the sensitivity and specificity of the existence of more than two colonized sites was only 73% and 50% respectively. Over a 6-month period, tri-weekly surveillance cultures identified colonization of more than two sites. In addition, DNA identification confirmed that the strains responsible for invasive infections were those that had previously colonized patients [94].

The colonization index is defined as the ratio of the number of sites colonized by *Candida* divided by the total number of sites tested. Its potential clinical value has been suggested in at least nine studies. Dubau et al reported that invasive candidiasis developed in only one of 35 surgical patients in whom empirical antifungals were prescribed when the index reached 0.5, and that it decreased rapidly in the other 34 patients [99]. Garbino et al, prospectively observed a decrease in the colonization index in a group of critically ill patients receiving antifungal prophylaxis [100]. Chabasse et al found a correlation between candiduria above 10^4 CFU / ml and a colonization index ≥ 0.5 [101]. Charles et al, have shown that colonization index values are significantly higher in medical patients than in surgical patients [102].

Duration of antibiotic exposure, haematological malignancy, candiduria and fungal colonization at entry predicted an increase in the colonization index. On the other hand, duration of exposure to antifungal agents was significantly associated with a decrease.

Normand et al, found a significant reduction in the colonization index in mechanically ventilated patients > 48 hours receiving oral nystatin prophylaxis [103]. Agvald-Öhman et al showed that a high colonization index after extensive gastro-abdominal surgery is closely associated with the development of invasive candidiasis [104]. Senn et al, reported a decrease in the colonization index in patients treated empirically with Caspofungin after gastrointestinal perforation, anastomotic leak or acute necrotizing pancreatitis [105].

3.1.2 Antibiotic therapy

Exposure to broad-spectrum antibiotic therapy is an important risk factor for the development of invasive candidiasis in both neutropenic and non-neutropenic patients [90].

Cephalosporins have a greater impact than other antibiotic classes [106]. The antibiotic's anti-anaerobic activity, broad antimicrobial spectrum and duration of exposure are closely linked to the risk of fungal complications [90].

According to Wey et al, the number of antibiotics used was one of the most important risk factors for candidemia [107]. In a study by Fraser et al, almost 94% of patients with candidemia had prior exposure to antibiotic therapy, and 61% had received more than four different agents [108].

3.1.3 Corticosteroid therapy

It induces immunosuppression by inhibiting the inflammatory response and cell-mediated immunity.

3.1.4 Chemotherapy

Antimitotics reduce the number of neutrophils, which play an important role in the innate *anti-Candida* defense by blocking filamentation and destroying yeasts through oxidative bursts.

Antimitotics also interfere with the complement system, resulting in reduced opsonin function.

3.1.5 Radiotherapy

It induces local immunodepression associated with dry mouth due to the destruction of the salivary glands.

3.1.6 Vascular approach

The vascular approach represents a risk factor for invasive candidiasis. Several studies have been carried out on this subject. Between 1988 and 1989, a study carried out in the United States at Barnes Hospital in Saint Louis showed a significant association between vascular access and the development of candidemia [107].

A one-year prospective observational study in western France showed that central venous catheters (CVCs) represent a second risk factor for candidemia: 72.6% of patients had a central venous catheter at the time of the candidemia episode, and 90 of these catheters were removed (66.7%), of which 77 were cultured, with positive results in 58.4% of cases [109].

Central venous catheters are a major risk factor for invasive candidiasis. In patients colonized with *Candida spp*, between 60% and 80% of candidemia episodes are secondary to vascular access infections. Indeed, catheter placement leads to adventitial trauma at the entry point, resulting in thrombosis. The thrombus will subsequently be colonized by yeasts that multiply in the vicinity of the catheter penetration point, leading to blood swarming and even fungal embolisms. Yeasts of the *Candida* genus, and more specifically *Candida parapsilosis*, have a particular affinity for the plastic material used in intravascular catheters, such as polyvinyl chloride [110].

3.1.7 Surgery

Abdominal surgery (gastrointestinal perforation, anastomotic ligation, liver transplantation, etc.) is a major risk factor, exposing surgical patients to high levels of colonization and/or invasive candidiasis [111].

3.1.8 Neutropenia

Neutrophils play an important role in the body's defense against fungal infections, and a severe ($<$ 500 cells//mm^3) and prolonged deficiency ($>$ 7 days) is the main risk factor for disseminated candidiasis [112].

In hematological malignancies such as myeloid or lymphoid leukemia, 20% to 50% of patients who die have clear signs of fungal invasion at autopsy [113].

Hematological malignancies can lead to neutropenia, as can cytostatic drugs or immunosuppressants used to prevent bone marrow transplant rejection in leukemia. Despite the initiation of antifungal treatment, the mortality rate remains high.

3.1.9 Severity scores

In order to express the severity of the pathology during the first 24 hours of admission to the intensive care unit, several severity scores need to be calculated. These scores integrate risk factors and colonization.

The main scores used are : APACHE (Acute Physiology and Chronic Health Evaluation), IGS (Indice de Gravité Simplifié) and MPM (Probability Mortality Model). The best-known are (Table II): the "Candida score", which takes into account the existence of severe sepsis, admission surgery, total parenteral nutrition and multifocal colonization. A score > 2.5 has a sensitivity of 81% and a specificity of 74%, requiring the initiation of early antifungal treatment [114], and the "Peritonitis score" takes into account the existence of shock on admission, a supramsocolic perforation, the existence of antibiotic therapy of more than 48 hours in progress, and female gender. A score ≥ 3 has a sensitivity of 84% and a specificity of 50%. [115].

Table. II: Candida score and Peritonitis score

Score	Presence of next item	Points
A. *Candida* score	Total parenteral nutrition	1
	Multiple *Candida* colonization	1
	Severe sepsis	2
	Surgery admission	1
B. Peritonitis score	Shock admission	1
	Supramesocolic perforation	1
	Female gender	1
	current antibiotic therapy ≥48 h	1

[Dupont H. Yeasts in intensive care. In: Sfar editor. Conférence d'actualisation. Congrès national d'anesthésie et de réanimation 2007; 415-32]

3.1.10 Extensive burns (> 50%)

Extensive burns destroy the first line of immune defense, exposing us to all kinds of micro-organism infections.

3.2 Minor risk factors

3.2.1 Ages extremes

The risk of *Candida* carriage and of developing severe invasive candidiasis increases in newborns and elderly subjects alike. This can be explained by the poor general condition of the elderly and the immaturity of the immune system in premature infants with a low birth weight of less than 1500g, which favours candidemia [7].

3.2.2 Length of stay

Length of stay is frequently described as a risk factor when it exceeds 7 days. In a study comparing a group of subjects with candidemia to a control group,

Wey et al found a significant difference between patients staying longer than seven days in a care unit and those with proven *Candida* infection [93].

3.2.3 Diabetes

It promotes genital and digestive candidiasis, without formal confirmation. Tissue glucose and lactate levels, with or without phagocytic deficiency, have been implicated.

3.2.4 Candiduria

Candiduria still poses interpretation problems, as urine is one of the most frequently colonized sites in the hospital environment. Indeed, the discovery of yeast in urine may indicate contamination, simple colonization or the first sign of an invasive infection [116]. According to a multicenter survey of intensive care units, significant candiduria in excess of 10^4 CFU/ml was associated with a colonization index≥ 0.5 [90].

Candidiasis is defined by the simple presence of yeasts in urocultures or on direct examination [117]. In other studies, quantification is a defining criterion; candiduria greater than or equal to 10^3 CFU/ml is sufficient for some [118,119] and greater than or equal to 10^4 CFU/ml for others [120,121]. Other authors agree on a value of at least 10^5 UFC/ml with signs of urinary tract infection [122].

Generally, candiduria is asymptomatic, and the most frequently incriminated factor is the urinary catheter, present in 77.6% of patients with candiduria.

4 PATHOPHYSIOLOGY OF SYSTEMIC CANDIDIASIS

Candida spp is an opportunistic pathogen with various virulence factors that facilitate colonization and invasion of host tissues. These virulence factors include morphological variability, the ability to produce hydrolytic enzymes and the ability to adhere via parietal adhesins (particularly mannoproteins) [123,124]. In order to colonize certain surfaces more easily, *Candida spp*, and *C. albicans* in particular, are able to form a biofilm on inert supports (catheters, probes, etc.). This is a complex structure combining yeast micro-colonies fixed by adhesins in a polymeric extracellular matrix, conferring greater resistance to antifungal agents [125,126].

Contamination is most often endogenous. *Candida albicans* are saprophytes of the digestive tract, and under the effect of favorable factors they proliferate in the digestive lumen, leading to a colonization phase. Once colonized, damaged mucosa allows microbial translocation across the intestinal digestive barrier, facilitated by conditions such as disruption of the mucosal barrier resulting from surgical procedures, intestinal pH-altering drugs and host immune deficiency [7] (Figure14).

Candida spp can initiate invasion of epithelial cells by two mechanisms: induction of endocytosis or active penetration of hyphae. The predominant mechanism in *C. albicans* is active invasion. Filaments physically disorganize cell structures. In addition, filamentation is accompanied by the co-regulated expression of hydrolases, leading to the alteration of host cells. This mechanism plays an important role in the invasion of deep tissues and blood vessels. After invasion, fungal elements reach the lumen of blood and lymphatic vessels.

The final stage is tissue multiplication in organs made accessible by the bloodstream.

More rarely, infection of a normally sterile site may occur after direct introduction of the pathogen (catheter infection, ascending renal candidiasis, peritonitis after intestinal surgery, manuportage) [127].

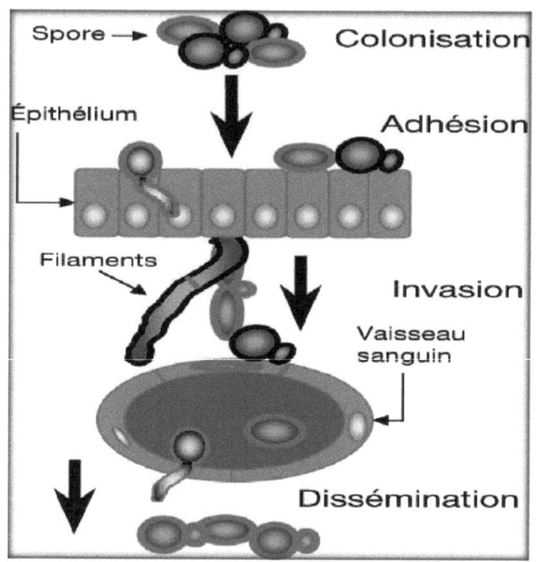

Figure. 14: Pathophysiology of *Candida* infections [7]

5 IMMUNITY AGAINST *CANDIDA* INFECTION

Candida spp is an opportunistic pathogen possessing a variety of virulence traits that facilitate colonization and invasion of host tissues and impairment of host defenses [128]. The establishment of a *Candida* infection in a susceptible host requires a well-coordinated series of events to bypass host immunity. Host defense mechanisms against candidiasis involve the activation of an acute inflammatory response by innate immunity, followed by specific T-cell-mediated or humoral B-cell-mediated immunity [129]. Although all branches of the host immune system are involved in the control of candidiasis, the predominance of the type of immunity strongly depends on the site and type of infection [130]. Innate immunity by neutrophil Polynuclei (NPCs) and macrophages plays a crucial role in protection against invasive *Candida* infections; the role of cell-mediated immunity (CMI) is well noted in the control of mucosal infections [130]. The role of antibody-mediated immunity (AMI) in candidiasis remains largely controversial [130].

The results of the interaction between the host immune system and *Candida spp* can lead either to elimination of the infectious pathogen, or to the development of a persistent infection such as chronic mucocutaneous candidiasis (CCMC) in the immunocompetent host, whereas candidemia and/or persistent systemic *Candida* infections are observed in the immunocompromised host [129].

5.1 Innate immunity

Physical and anatomical barriers such as skin and mucosal surfaces, which limit the entry of pathogens into host tissue, are considered the host's first line of defense against infection.

Normal skin produces multiple substances such as free fatty acids that inhibit the growth and multiplication *of Candida spp* [131].

Epithelial cells secrete cytokines and inhibitory chemokines that gradually diffuse to their surface and prevent yeast cell adhesion [130].

Endothelial cells can phagocytose *Candida* cells [130].

Various mechanisms control the proliferation of *Candida spp* in the gastrointestinal tract. Salivary flow prevents yeast adhesion to mucosal surfaces [132]. The flow and composition of saliva prevents oropharyngeal candidiasis in healthy individuals by maintaining a dynamic balance between *Candida spp* and other commensal flora [133].

A variety of non-specific antimicrobial factors present in saliva contribute to innate immunity against *Candida spp*. These include Lysozyme, lactoperoxidase histatins, calprotectin and lactoferrin [133].

Lactoferrin acts as a chelating agent that competes with oral microorganisms for free ionic radicals, which are essential for bacterial and fungal proliferation. In addition, it destroys the fungal cell wall and activates intracellular autolytic enzymes [133].

Histatin proteins exhibit broad-spectrum antifungal activity against pathogenic fungi such as *Candida spp, Cryptococcus neoformans* and *Aspergillus fumigatus* [133]. Edgerton et al have reported the *anti-Candida* activity of histatin 5; when internalized by *Candida*, the latter leads to several deleterious effects such as damage to mitochondria and cytoplasmic membrane, efflux of ATP and other nucleotides, resulting in cell death [134,135].

Calprotectin is a calcium- and zinc-binding protein produced by polynuclear cells, monocytes, macrophages and mucosal keratinocytes. It blocks *Candida* growth by depriving the yeast of zinc [133].

The commensal bacterial flora of the gastrointestinal tract inhibits *Candida* proliferation by various mechanisms such as nutritional and ecological competition at the site of adhesion [131]. Of the various mechanisms responsible for the control of *Candida* by commensal flora, competition for nutrition is the most important [136]. Depletion of the commensal bacterial flora by broad-spectrum antibiotics is one of the risk factors for candidiasis [131,136].

Once *Candida spp* penetrate the gastrointestinal mucosa and gain access to host tissue, a series of serum factors are activated. *Candida* surface proteins strongly stimulate the 3 complement activation pathways (classical, alternative and mannose binding lectin (MBL) [136]. Complement activation leads to opsonization and intracellular destruction of *Candida spp.*

The alternative complement pathway, activated by *Candida spp* cell wall components, is primarily responsible for phagocytosis of yeast cells [131].

The mannose binding lectin (MBL) cascade plays an important role in opsonization, phagocytosis and other complement functions.

The C3b and C3d fragments are both capable of binding to *C. Albicans* [131].

The interaction between activated C3b and the complement receptor CR3 facilitates phagocytosis of *Candida* cells. C5 also plays an important role in immunity to *Candida* infections. Activation of C5 triggers the formation of C5b, which facilitates phagocytosis and the release of terminal complement components [137]. Complement deficiency leads to poor host resistance to candidiasis.

Neutrophils play a vital role in host defense against invasive candidiasis [130]. This is demonstrated by the high incidence of systemic *Candida* infections such as candidemia in patients with prolonged neutropenia or neutrophil disorders [138]. Neutrophils are the only immunocytes that block the transition of *Candida spp* from the yeast to the filamentous form [137]. This type of leukocyte also controls the elimination of *Candida spp* from the bloodstream.

Among the mechanisms responsible for the destruction of *Candida* by PNNs, the "oxidative burst" seems to be the most important. The oxidative burst is the process of rapid formation of reactive oxygen intermediates [137,139]. This process requires assembly of the NADPH-oxidase enzyme complex in the cytoplasmic complex or membrane phagosome to release superoxide [137,139].

Natural killer (NK) cells are another host defense mechanism against candidiasis. NK cell activity is largely due to the production of granulocyte macrophage colony stimulating Factor (GM-CSF). NK cells are also responsible for activating phagocytic mononuclear cells (MPCs) and PNNs.

The ability of PNNs and CPMs to phagocytose *Candida* cells does not mean that they necessarily destroy the yeast. Although phagocytes are capable of killing most yeast cells and hyphae, some yeasts escape this process and proliferate in phagocytes. Mechanisms such as inhibition of reactive oxygen production, prevention of phagolysosome fusion and pH increase are responsible for protecting yeast from phagocytosis [140]. In addition, the transformation of yeast into filamentous form in the cytoplasm of immune cells inhibits mitosis and leads to apoptotosis [140].

5.2 Cell-mediated immunity (CMI)

Cell-mediated immunity plays an important role in preventing mucosal candidiasis. Patients with T-cell deficiencies: (HIV, transplant recipients and those on corticosteroid therapy) are at high risk of developing mucosal candidiasis, but rarely develop disseminated candidiasis [140].

A strong correlation has been observed between oropharyngeal candidiasis (COP) and the reduction of CD4 + cells in the blood. In HIV-infected individuals, the depletion of CD4+ cells below a critical threshold of 200 cells/mm3 usually triggers the onset of COP [133].

Mucocutaneous *Candida spp* overgrowth can also occur in patients with idiopathic CD4 lymphocytopenia or after anti-CD52 monoclonal therapy [136].

Type 1 (Th1) T-helper cells confer protection against candidiasis, while Th2 responses lack the ability to inhibit fungal growth and multiplication, thus increasing susceptibility to infection. Consequently, a shift from Th1 to Th2 in the peripheral circulation may increase the risk of COP [130].

Candida cell wall components such as mannan and β-1,3-D-glucan are pathogenic molecules (PAMPs) recognized by phagocyte surface receptors (PRRs) [129]. These receptors (PRRs) are grouped into several families such as Toll-like receptors (TLRs), C-type lectin receptors (CLRs) and the leucine-rich nucleotide-binding domain (NLR) [129].

The interaction between PAMPs and PRRs induces Th differentiation into Th 17[136]. Cytokines (IL-17 and IL-22) secreted by Th 17, trigger the production of an antimicrobial peptide known as β-defensins. The latter controls *Candida* proliferation. The release of IL-17 and IL-22 also recruits and activates neutrophils, leading to the elimination of *Candida* infection [141].

IL-22 plays a vital role in limiting fungal growth and maintaining epithelial barrier function.

5.3 Humoral immunity

Although different classes of antibodies such as IgG, IgM or IgA are (except in highly immunosuppressed patients) produced in all clinical forms of candidiasis, the protective role of humoral immunity is largely unknown. In fact, patients with mucosal candidiasis show normal or high levels of *anti-Candida* antibodies [130]. To date, there are no studies demonstrating direct evidence of increased susceptibility to mucocutaneous disease and systemic candidiasis in patients with B-cell abnormalities (either congenital or acquired).

IgG and IgM are found in the sera of patients with mucocutaneous candidiasis and deep-lying candidiasis. Moreover, these antibodies can also be observed during asymptomatic colonization at low titres. Few previous studies have reported an increase in salivary IgA and IgG in patients with candidiasis.

Anti-mannan and anti-glucan antibodies have been demonstrated in serum. However, their protective role is uncertain, as high levels of these antibodies are observed in infections with a poor prognosis [142].

Coogan et al (1994) observed an increase in salivary antibodies in AIDS patients compared with controls. They suggested that in an HIV-infected individual, antibody titer appears to reflect responses to *Candida* rather than protection. These salivary immunoglobulins are thought to interfere *with Candida* adhesion to the salivary mucosa. However, this mechanism breaks down with increasing yeast cell load [143].

6 CLINIC

Systemic or invasive candidiasis are infections caused by yeasts of the *Candida* genus. This definition covers candidemia and deep-rooted visceral candidiasis, most often originating in hematogenous dissemination.

Candidemia defines a situation where *Candida* has been identified by at least one blood culture. Deep visceral candidiasis corresponds to a situation where a yeast has been identified in several non-contiguous sites, implying hematogenous dissemination, although blood cultures are sometimes negative.

There is no specific symptomatology for candidemia and deep-rooted candidiasis :

- Irregular, antibiotic-resistant fever.
- Altered general condition is observed in around 80% of cases.
- Leukocytosis in 50% of cases.

Candidemia that is detected late or goes undetected has a high risk of uni- or multivisceral localization, which may come to the fore weeks after the first episode.

In 10% of cases, systemic candidiasis may manifest as skin lesions (Figure 15) in the form of well-demarcated maculopapular, maculonodular or red purpura lesions, located on the trunk and limbs, or even covering the entire body [38]. These cutaneous localizations appear early in the sepsis phase and may be the first visible sign of deep-seated candidiasis. After direct examination and culture of the skin fragments, a skin biopsy can confirm the candidal origin of the lesions.

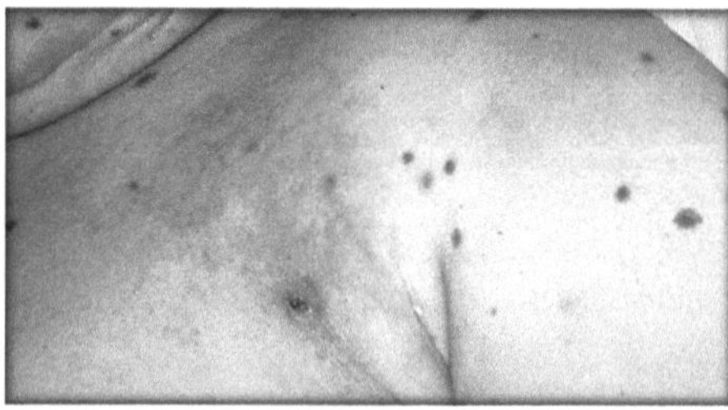

Figure. 15: Skin lesions at the heart of *Candida sp* septicemia p [22]

Ocular manifestations should also be systematically sought in cases of candidemia.

Finally, other, rarer localizations of disseminated candidiasis may exist, such as cardiac, renal, meningeal, pulmonary, pancreatic, hepatosplenic, osteoarticular and neurological.

6.1   retinal lesions [144]

Two metastatic ocular anomalies may be observed in the course of candidemia. These are endophthalmitis with vitritis, usually presenting as fluffy balls extending into the vitreous body (Figure 16), and chorioretinitis, with abnormalities limited to the chorioretinal layers.

The extent of ocular lesions depends on the stage at which candidemia is diagnosed. At first, lesions are localized, and in the absence of antifungal treatment, full-blown endophthalmitis occurs. However, antifungal treatment limits ocular manifestations, and progression to endophthalmitis is rare.

To date, retinal lesions during candidemia have been described in small cohorts of patients. Only two studies have investigated ocular lesions during candidemia; the authors found *Candida* in chorioretinitis in 2% - 9% and in endophthalmitis in 1% of cases.

Ocular candidiasis is treated with systemic or intavitreal injections of an antifungal agent, sometimes combined with vitrectomy. Systemic amphotericin B and echinocandins do not penetrate the vitreous humor well, while fluconazole and voriconazole reach vitreous concentrations of between 25% and 100% of their serum concentrations.

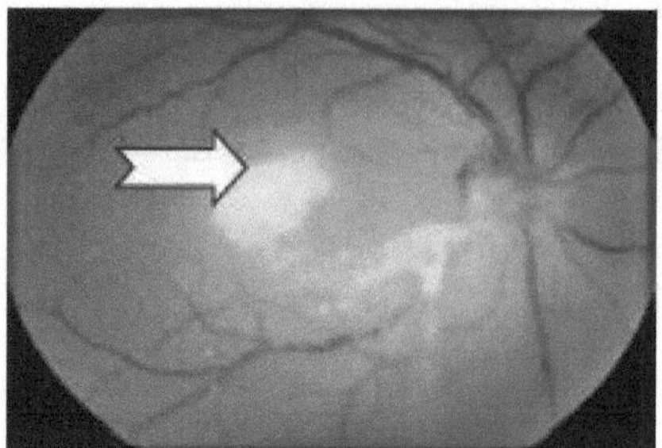

Figure. 16: Fundus of *Candida* endophthalmitis (Lint ball appearance) [145]

6.2   Renal candidiasis

According to autopsy data, *Candida* pyelonephritis is the consequence of candidemia originating from a distant infection, and is only observed in immunocompromised patients [146]. Renal involvement is observed in 80% of cases of systemic candidiasis [147]. In 1963, Hurley et al experimentally demonstrated that the presence of *Candida* in the blood inevitably leads to its presence in the kidney [148].

Renal involvement begins with cortical damage, which may extend to the renal papillae, causing necrotic lesions and micro-abscesses.

The formation of fungal aggregates known as "Fungus balls" or "bezoars" has occurred in the urinary tract in the renal pelvis, ureter and bladder [149,150] (Figure 17).

Clinically, candidal pyelonephritis is identical to bacterial pyelonephritis, manifesting as: fever, chills, lumbar or lumbo-abdominal pain. Less frequent symptomatic forms include renal colic, acute obstruction [151], papillary necrosis [152] and renal failure.

Its prognosis is sometimes severe when the papillae are involved, with suppuration of the renal parenchyma.

Complications may arise in the absence of treatment, such as parenchymal micro-abscesses (visible on CT scan) that can lead to renal failure.

Candidiasis is present, but cannot be used on its own as a diagnostic criterion. It is difficult to distinguish simple colonization from true infection.

Renal infection can also have a retrograde origin, favored by the presence of a urinary catheter or diabetes.

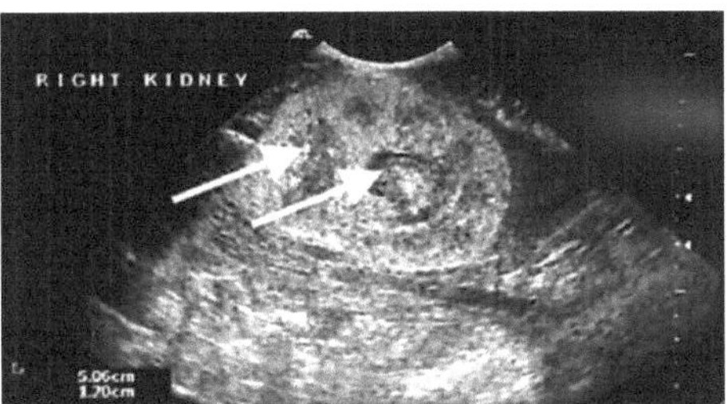

Figure. 17: Renal Fugus balls (Bezoard) [153]

6.3   Cardiac candidiasis

Fungal endocarditis remains the most serious form of infective endocarditis, with *Candida albicans* responsible for 24-46% of all cases of fungal endocarditis and 3.4% of all cases of valvular prosthetic endocarditis, with a mortality rate of around 50% [154,155].

It is very difficult to diagnose and treat [156]. It is generally diagnosed post-mortem [157].

The cardiac sites affected in neonates differ significantly from those of adults (mitral or aortic valve), with the right atrium predominating in 63% of neonates [158].

Among the most common risk factors for the development of fungal endocarditis are : Previous surgery and intravenous drug use. Other risk factors included parenteral nutrition, immunosuppression, underlying cardiac anomalies, prosthetic heart valves, indwelling central venous catheters, prolonged use of broad-spectrum antibiotics and cardiovascular surgery, progression of myelodysplastic syndrome, use of steroidal and cytotoxic drugs and bone marrow transplantation with high-dose immunosuppressive therapy [159].

Symptoms are similar to those of bacterial endocarditis: fever, purpura, splenomegaly, murmur. However, echocardiography reveals larger vegetations, which can lead to serious arterial embolism. Ellis et al reported that the sensitivity of transthoracic and transoesophageal echocardiography techniques specifically focused on fungal endocarditis reached 77% [160]. Transthoracic echocardiography provides an accurate diagnosis of fungal endocarditis, identifying 89% of vegetations. Histopathological examination of the vegetative tissue revealed a large fungal mass around the vegetation site with no infiltration of inflammatory cells [161].

Precise molecular methods were available for the diagnosis of many infections, which were up to three times more sensitive than Gram stain and culture. Badiee et al, reported that polymerase chain reaction was positive in all tissue samples and in 10/11 blood samples [154].

The European Society of Clinical Microbiology and Infectious Diseases (ESCMID) recommends that patients with infective endocarditis undergoing surgical treatment should receive antifungal therapy for the management of *Candida* disease.

The molecules used are liposomal amphotericin B for one week or caspofungin for 8 weeks, with or without additional flucytosine, followed by fluconazole [162].

Candida pericarditis is a rare but serious condition that can lead to severe sepsis, tamponade and even death if not diagnosed and treated in time. Clinical signs are often subtle and non-specific. However, any unexplained fever accompanied by pleural effusion in a patient at high risk of systemic candidiasis points to the diagnosis [163].

Candida myocarditis is rarely detected antemortem. Its incidence is therefore poorly understood. It can occur as an extension of endocarditis, or as microabscesses disseminated in the myocardium during a systemic form.

6.4 Hepatosplenic candidiasis

Hepatosplenic candidiasis is the most common form of chronic disseminated candidiasis. It typically occurs in patients with long-term neutropenia lasting more than 10 days and less than 500 cells/ mm^3 [164].

Clinically, hepatosplenic candidiasis is strongly suggested by persistent fever despite normalization of neutrophil levels. Other non-specific symptoms may be associated, such as abdominal pain, diarrhea, tenderness, nausea, vomiting and sometimes jaundice, which is present in at least a third of patients [165]. Serum alkaline phosphatase levels are three times higher with other liver function tests, in particular transaminases and gamma-glutamyl-transferase being less sensitive [165].

In hepatosplenic candidiasis, blood cultures are often negative [165]. A possible explanation for the low blood culture yield may be hematogenous dissemination limited to the venous portal system. In a series from Italy, two-thirds of cases had *Candida-positive* biopsies [165]. However, hepatosplenic candidiasis becomes clinically apparent only with resolution neutropenia and thrombocytopenia. If chronic disseminated candidiasis is impossible to prove by microbiological evidence, we may routinely perform a biopsy. Imaging is particularly important in defining probable hepatosplenic candidiasis [166].

Computed tomography (CT) or magnetic resonance imaging (MRI) rarely detects hepatosplenic candidiasis before bone marrow reconstitution and recovery from neutropenia [167]. The most sensitive phase or CT is the acute or arterial dominant phase, 25-35 seconds after contrast injection, showing a hyperdense rim surrounding a hypodense "bull's eye" center (Figure. 18). In the portal venous phase, i.e. 60-80 seconds after injection, microabscesses in the form of hypodense lesions $\leq$ 1 cm in size may appear (Figure. 19).

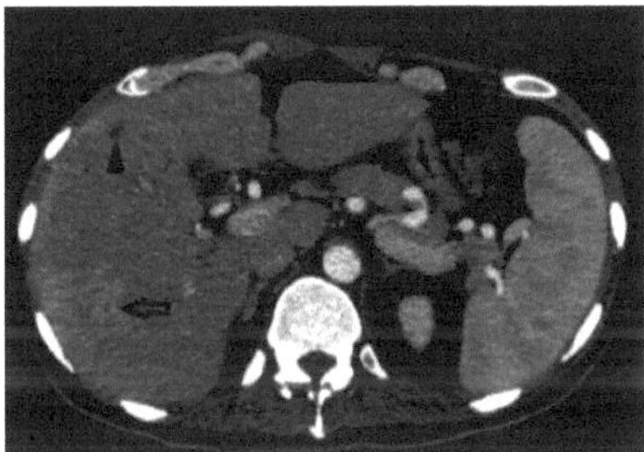

Figure. 18: Abdominal CT scan in the arterial contrast phase showing a hyperdense border surrounding a hypodense "bull's eye" center[164].

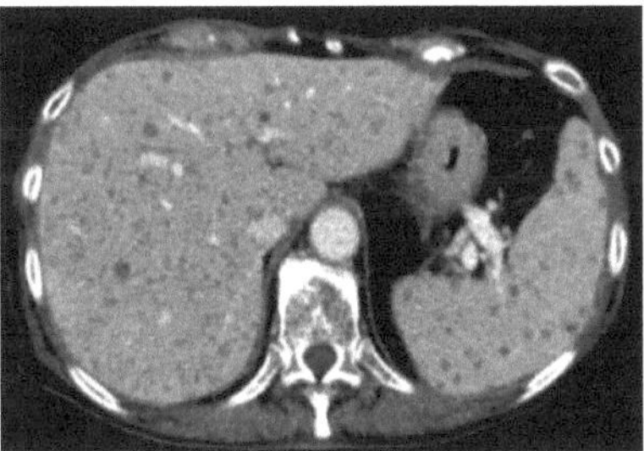

Figure. 19: Abdominal CT in portal venous phase with multiple hypodense lesions in liver and spleen (micro abscesses)[164]

6.5 Peritoneal candidiasis

Peritoneal candidiasis is relatively rare compared with bacterial peritonitis, and is associated with significant morbidity and mortality [168]. According to some recent series, 3-6% of dialysis-related episodes of peritonitis are caused by *Candida* [168,169].

Candida peritonitis is associated with significantly higher rates of hospitalization, and transfer to permanent hemodialysis [170]. Previous episodes of bacterial peritonitis on broad-spectrum antibacterial therapy are a risk factor for peritoneal candidiasis.

The clinical picture is atypical, and the infecting organism may be difficult to isolate. In contrast to other forms of deep candidiasis, dissemination is markedly infrequent. Peritoneal candidiasis is strongly suspected when a patient treated for bacterial peritonitis fails to respond to antibacterial therapy within 3 to 4 days. Peritoneal dialysate typically contains neutrophilic polynuclear cells, but sometimes lymphocytes predominate. Gram staining of dialysate can reveal the microorganism involved. Many clinical reports stress the importance of catheter removal for recovery [168, 169,170].

Intraperitoneal instillation of amphotericin B is no longer recommended, as it is associated with chemical peritonitis and the development of peritoneal fibrosis. Antifungal regimens are similar to those recommended for candidemia [171].

6.6 Biliary candidiasis

This infection is usually diagnosed after surgery or invasive procedures of the biliary tract. In a series of 123 consecutive patients undergoing endoscopic retrograde cholangiopancreatography for various indications, *Candida* was found in 44% of bile samples [172]. Another presentation is alithiasic cholecystitis in critically ill or immunocompromised patients with disseminated candidiasis, a condition associated with high mortality [173].

Although isolation of *Candida* from biliary sources is insufficient evidence of a pathogenic role, the organism has been implicated in acute cholecystitis, including gangrenous cholecystitis and cholangitis. *Candida* cholangitis has been reported in patients with biliary and malignant obstruction of the bile ducts.

6.7 Pancreatic candidiasis

Pancreatic candidiasis accounts for 5 - 68% of severe pancreatitis [174, 175,176]. It is most often associated with prolonged hospitalization, multi-organ failure and increased mortality in patients with severe pancreatitis [175,176].

Pancreatic candidiasis is often a complication of pancreatic injury or surgery. Prolonged placement of indwelling devices for pancreatic fluid collection further increases the risk. Evidence of the importance of *Candida* in pancreatic infection processes continues to mount. The presence of *Candida* in pancreatic cultures, particularly in drains or mixed flora, has often been overlooked. However, isolation of the organism from pancreatic necrotic tissue should generally be considered significant [174,175].

Diagnosis is made by culturing samples obtained from pancreatic or peripancreatic necrosis, abscesses and pseudocysts obtained during surgery, endoscopic necrosectomy or catheter-guided aspiration. Ultimately, histopathological confirmation of tissue invasion is the only convincing evidence of pancreatic candidiasis.

Drainage and debridement of infected necrosis are important for the eradication of *Candida* from poorly perfused tissue, where antifungal agents may not reach therapeutic levels. Drainage of small abscesses or pseudocysts infected with *Candida* has been effective in some cases. Systemic antifungal therapy should be initiated early in the course of the disease.

A clear association between death and lack of antifungal treatment in a series of 13 patients with acute necrotizing pancreatitis and pancreatic *Candida* infection has been reported [176].

6.8 Pulmonary candidiasis

Yeasts of the *Candida* genus can infect the lung in two ways: by aspiration of infected oropharyngeal secretions (primary pneumonitis) or by direct invasion during sepsis (secondary pneumonitis).

Candida-positive lung samples do not distinguish between colonization and nosocomial bronchopulmonary infection.

Numerous studies have described nosocomial *Candida* pneumonia in a variety of circumstances. In 1995, the EPIC study, a prevalence survey of nosocomial infection in intensive care units, reported a rate of 46.9% of pneumopathies, 14% of which were related to yeasts, mainly of the *Candida* genus [92]. Nosocomial *Candida* pneumonitis has also been reported in diabetics and alcoholics, patients in whom yeast colonization of the mouth and throat is common [177,178].

In these patients, the criteria for diagnosing *Candida* pneumonia are the usual ones, i.e. tracheal aspiration or distal swabs protected above the positivity thresholds. The shared presence of immunodepression, hospitalization in intensive care or post-operative care is a risk factor for nosocomial pneumopathy. *Candida* pneumonia in cancer patients undergoing chemotherapy, organ transplants or HIV infection is a marker of severely impaired immune defenses and particular susceptibility to opportunistic infections [179].

Symptomatology is atypical, with fever, polypnoea, cough with sputum and sometimes chest pain [179].

Pneumonitis secondary to hematogenous dissemination presents as diffuse parenchymal involvement, but clinical symptoms are usually masked by other manifestations of invasive candidiasis.

Diagnosis is very difficult, rarely confirmed antemortem, radiological examination has no specificity, and the positivity of alveolar lavage is of no real value. Biopsy is the only diagnostic criterion to be taken into consideration [179].

6.9 Cerebrospinal candidiasis

Candida infection of the meninges is the most common infection of the central nervous system (CNS). However, intracranial abscesses can occur either in isolation or in association with meningitis [180,181].

Abscesses are usually small micro-abscesses, multiple, and associated with disseminated infection in immunocompromised hosts[181].

Candida meningitis may appear as a manifestation of disseminated candidiasis, which occurs most often in premature neonates, in the presence of ventricular drainage devices [182]. Hematogenous spread of *Candida* may occur at the time of craniotomy (or via a ventricular shunt). Clinically, a classic meningeal syndrome may be observed, but diagnosis remains difficult as changes in cerebrospinal fluid (CSF) cytology and chemistry are not constant. More frequently, pleocytosis with lymphocyte predominance, increased protein levels and moderate hypoglycorachia are observed. Culture isolation of *Candida* is rarely positive.

6.10 Oteo-articular candidiasis

Osteoarticular *Candida* infections are most often due to hematogenous seeding of the joint or bone in patients who have been candidemic.

The areas most often infected during an episode of candidemia in adults are the intervertebral discs and knee joints.

Exogenous inoculation can also lead to infection after trauma or at the time of intra-articular injection (most often the knee) or prosthesis implantation [183].

7 BIOLOGICAL DIAGNOSIS

Invasive candidiasis remains a serious infection with a high mortality rate, despite the availability of new antifungal agents. This mortality is largely due to the difficulty of establishing an early diagnosis, and therefore the need for early treatment.

Biological diagnosis of invasive candidiasis relies firstly on direct examination of biological products, to identify the presence of budding yeasts with or without *Candida* mycelia. At the same time, a culture on specific medium(s) is performed to isolate the micro-organism. The next step is to identify the *Candida* species involved, using conventional techniques (biochemical and immunological tests) or new technologies (molecular biology).

Indirect techniques (antibody and antigen testing) are invaluable for diagnosing invasive candidiasis.

Antifungal susceptibility testing will only be considered in certain circumstances (deep-rooted or recurrent infections, prior exposure to azole antifungals).

7.1 Direct diagnosis and identification

Mycological diagnosis of candidiasis begins with direct examination of the sample, whether superficial or deep, followed by culture to isolate the germ(s) present. Isolated yeast colonies can then be identified on the basis of morphological, immunological, biochemical and, if necessary, genotypic criteria [184, 185,186].

7.1.1 Withdrawals

Diagnosis of mycosis depends on the quality and quantity of a sample being collected in a sterile container. Samples must be sent immediately to the laboratory; otherwise, they are stored at +4°C. Mucocutaneous samples should preferably be taken by the biologist himself, and at a distance from any local or general antifungal treatment.

7.1.2 Direct examination

Direct examination (DE) is the first step in the laboratory, enabling rapid diagnosis and treatment. It consists of looking for budding yeasts, with or without filaments.

Direct examination is carried out either directly in the fresh state, by mounting in a non-colored liquid (distilled water or sterile physiological water), or using a dye that enhances visualization of the blastoconidia: 2% lugol, toluidine blue, lactophenol blue, chlorazole black or congo red.

Deep-site samples (bronchoalveolar lavage fluid (BALF), pleural fluid, joint fluid, tissue biopsies, etc.) are spread on slides. Smears are fixed with heat or alcohol, then stained with May-Grunwald-Giemsa (MGG), or treated with silver impregnation (Gomori-Grocott or Musto techniques).

Anatomopathological examination is essential for diagnosing deep-seated mycoses. The stains used are Schiff's periodic acid (PAS), Gomori-Grocott silver impregnation and hematein-eosin-safran (HES).

7.1.3 Crops

Yeasts of the *Candida* genus are undemanding, and Sabouraud agar medium supplemented with chloramphenicol and/or gentamicin plus cycloheximide (Actidione) is traditionally the most widely used. Petri dishes offer a larger inoculation surface than tubes. On the other hand, the risk of contamination by airborne filamentous fungal spores is greater, and the media dry out more quickly. Incubation takes place at 37°C. Incubation time is adapted to the type of sample. An incubation period of 24 to 72 hours is generally sufficient to isolate the majority of *Candida*, but it can be as long as one to four weeks.

Candida colonies appear after 24 to 48 hours incubation at 37°C and measure a few millimeters in diameter. Rather whitish in color, their surface is smooth, shiny and glossy.

Other culture media are used, to which chromogenic substances are added, giving the colonies that develop there a particular coloration, which varies according to the species. In most cases, this staining is based on the detection of hexosaminidase-type enzymatic activity (N-acetyl-α-D-galactosaminidase).

All these environments at least allow direct identification of :

- *Candida albicans*, with colonies staining blue (Candida ID® 2, bioMerieux) (Candichrom®, ELITech Microbio; ChromID®, bioMerieux), green (CHROMagar® Candida, Becton- Dickinson; OCCA®, Oxoid) or violet-pink (CandiSelect® 4, Bio-Rad).

- *C. dubliniensis* develops a coloration very similar to that of *C. albicans* on these different media. Differentiation between these two species then requires specific tests.

- *C. tropicalis, C. glabrata* and *C. krusei* form blue colonies of different appearance on CandiSelect® 4 medium.

- *C. tropicalis, C. lusitaniae* and *C. kefyr* form pink colonies on Candida ID®2

- *C tropicalis* forms bluish colonies on OCCA® medium.

- *C. krusei* irregular pink colonies on OCCA® medium.

- On CHROMagar® Candida, *C. tropicalis* forms metallic blue colonies and C. krusei rather rough, pale pink colonies.

CHROMagar® medium (Figure 20) therefore offers the broadest spectrum for direct colony identification [187].

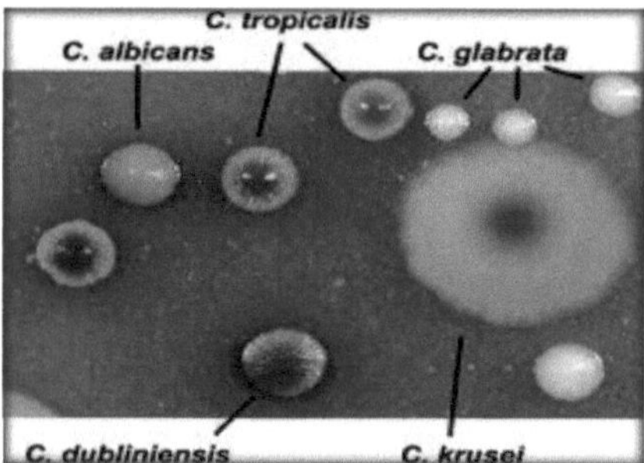

Figure. 20: Appearance of different *Candida* species on CHROMagar Candida medium [188].

Candida albicans fluoresces bluish when cultured on Fluoroplate® Candida medium (Merck), and colonies are observed under ultraviolet light at 366 nm [189]. The need for specific equipment limits the use of this medium.

7.1.4 Blood cultures

For blood cultures, it is preferable to use a specific medium promoting fungal growth (Bactec® IC/F Mycosis, Becton-Dickinson), as well as an automated reading system based on the measurement of CO_2 released during yeast growth (Bactec®, Becton-Dickinson; BacT/ALERT®, bioMerieux). Detection of fungal growth is based on automatic colorimetric (BacT/ALERT®) or fluormetric (Bactec®) measurements;

prior use of the Isolator® system (lysis-centrifugation) shortens the time between inoculation and detection of fungal growth [190].

According to ESCMID, the recommended total number of blood cultures is 3, with a total volume of 40-60 ml for adults, divided into 3 aerobic and 3 anaerobic vials with 10 ml each. Blood cultures should be taken successively (30 min) from different sites. Incubation time 2-5 days [162].

In the event of a positive result, it is necessary to perform a subculture on standard and/or chromogenic media in order to identify the fungus and determine its sensitivity to antifungal agents. and/or chromogenic media to identify the fungus and determine its sensitivity to antifungal agents.

7.1.5 Identification

In current practice, identification of the various *Candida* species is based on morphological, physiological and, more recently, immunological characteristics [185]. Mass spectrometry and molecular biology, although promising, are currently only used by specialized centers and research teams.

7.1.5.1 *Candida albicans*

Candida albicans is the species most frequently isolated and considered the most virulent. Historically, a number of tests were developed in the 1960s-1970s, and in their day represented reference methods [191, 192].

These are :

➢ Blastesis test (germination or filamentation)

- Performed by incubating the isolate for 3 to 4 hours in serum at 35-37°C. *Candida albicans* is then identified by the production of a thin germ tube of homogeneous diameter with no constriction at its base, emerging from the mother cell.

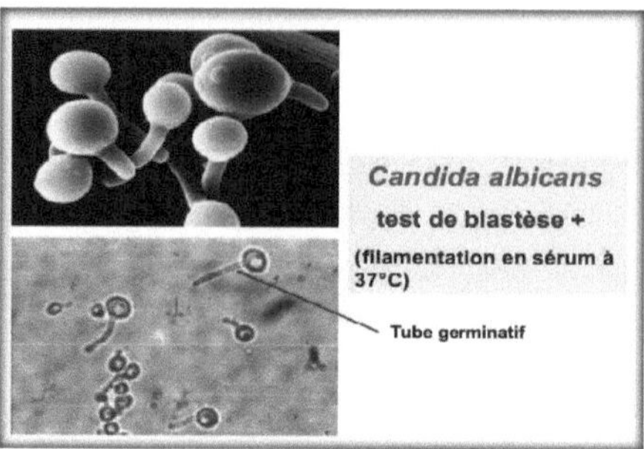

Figure. 21: Positive blasting test (Filamentation) (*Candida albicans*) [193]

➢ The chlamydosporulation test

Based on a 24 to 48-hour culture at 25-28°C of the deep streak isolate in PCB (potato, carrot, bile) or RAT (rice, agar, tween 80) medium. *Candida albicans* is identified by the production of Chlamydospores, rounded structures 10 to 15µm in diameter with thick walls (double-contour appearance) produced singly or in clusters at the tip of the pseudomycelium.

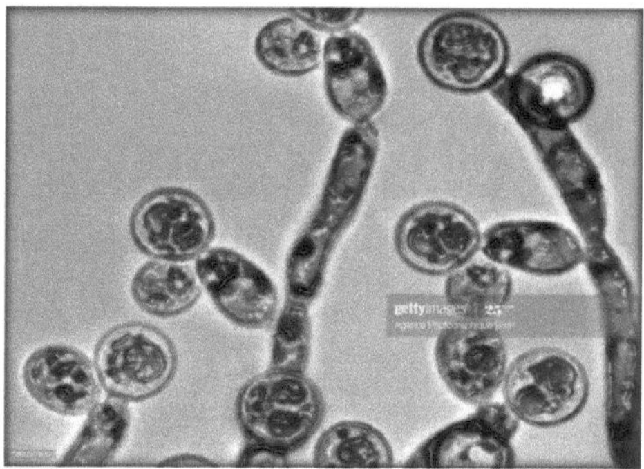

Figure. 22: Positive Chlamydosporulation test [194]

On the other hand, these two tests do not allow true differentiation between *Candida dubliniensis* and *Candida albicans*, and have been advantageously replaced by more rapid and/or species-specific tests.

➢ Immunological test

Bichrolatex®albicans (Fumouze Diagnostics) is based on the principle of on-slide coagglutination of coloured latex particles sensitized with a monoclonal antibody recognizing a *C. albicans* parietal antigen [195]. A positive test results in the appearance of red agglutinates on a green background; freshly isolated colonies are identified within minutes as *C. albicans* or *C. dubliniensis*. Differentiation between these two species then relies on a second device, the bichrodubli® (Fumouze Diagnostics) [196].

➢ Metabolic test

Three devices are currently on the market: Murex C. albicans® (Murex Diagnostics), Albicans-Sure® (Clinical Standards Laboratories) and BactiCard Candida® (Remel CO). All three tests involve the detection of dual β-galactosaminidase and L-proline aminopeptidase activity, positive only for *C. albicans* colonies [197].

7.1.5.2 *Non-albicans* species

➢ Reduction of tetrazolium salts

This technique is based on the reduction of 2,3,5-triphenyltetrazolium chloride, incorporated into the culture medium, to an insoluble colored product that gives *Candida* colonies a coloration ranging from white to red, depending on the species.

➢ Immunological tests

These tests are performed on isolated colonies and give a result in just a few minutes. Latex particle agglutination reagents are still used, such as Krusei color® for *C. krusei* and Bichrodubli® for *C. dubliniensis* (Fumouze Diagnostics) [196,198].

➢ Enzyme tests

The Glabrata RTT® test (Fumouze Diagnostics) specifically identifies *Candida glabrata* colonies [199]. This test is based on the ability of *Candida glabrata* to hydrolyze trehalose and not maltose. It uses a glucose oxidase to identify the glucose formed from each of these two carbohydrates. The result is obtained in 15 minutes.

➢ Biochemical tests

A wide range of galleries are available. The vast majority are based on the study of carbohydrate assimilation (auxanogram) and fermentation (zymogram).

[200].

7.1.6 Determining sensitivity to antifungal agents

Antifungal susceptibility testing enables us to study the sensitivity of isolated strains to the various antifungal agents available, and if possible to determine their minimum inhibitory concentrations (MICs). It can be used to guide antifungal therapy, as well as to monitor the emergence of resistant strains.

There are two reference techniques: CLSI (Clinical and Laboratory Standards Institute) and EUCAST (European Committee on Anti-microbial Susceptibility). As these methods are not commercially available, they are performed only by reference centers. The European technique, developed after the American one, was designed to standardize the reading of results (spectrophotometric measurement instead of visual reading) and shorten the reading time (24 instead of 48 hours) [201].

A commonly used test (**Etest®**) is an antifungal strip method. The reverse side of the strips is impregnated with a continuous, exponential gradient of antifungal agent; the front side is graduated, representing a concentration scale enabling MIC readings (µg/ml). This technique, which first appeared in the 1990s, was initially used as an antibiotic susceptibility testing technique, but was soon adapted to antifungal agents [201].

7.2 Indirect diagnosis

Since fungal blood cultures have a low sensitivity (50%) and therefore a low yield. This observation has led to a search for other diagnostic aids. Currently, immunological methods are being developed to detect markers of invasive fungal infection, such as serum antibodies or circulating antigens, which are often used as complementary tests.

7.2.1 Test for *anti-Candida* serum antibodies

Different techniques use soluble antigens (HAI, IEP, ES, ELISA), or figured antigens (IFI). A distinction is traditionally made between screening techniques (IFI, HAI and ELISA) and confirmatory techniques (IEP, ES). The positivity of a screening technique must be verified by a confirmatory technique. It is also recommended to combine at least two techniques.

The tests currently on the market are listed below:

- Indirect immunofluorescence (IFI) uses C. albicans blastospores, which are deposited on ready-to-use glass slides (Candida-Spot IF®, bioMerieux).
- Indirect hemagglutination (HAI) detects IgG or IgM antibodies (Candidose Fumouze®, Fumouze Diagnostics).
- ELISA tests for antibodies to parietal mannans (Platelia® Candida Ab (Bio-Rad); Serion® ELISA classic Candida albicans IgG/IgM/IgA, (Virion/Serion).
- Immunoelectrophoresis (IEP) and electrosyneresis (ES) detect precipitating antibodies (C. albicans antigens, Bio-Rad) and enable semi-quantitative assessment (number of arcs and intensity). It is thus possible to judge the evolution of a patient's antibody titer by having different sera migrate side by side with a reference serum.

Candidiasis serology is of limited value in immunocompromised patients. Indeed, patients with neutropenia should be monitored serologically as soon as they are admitted, in addition to testing for circulating antigens. Optimal use of the tests requires bi-weekly determination of antibody titres, and follow-up of titres during the course of the infection.

Other techniques rely on the detection of antibodies directed against mycelial antigens present in invasive candidiasis, 48 kDa anti-vacuolar enolase antibodies, or antibodies directed against the 47 kDa subunit of Heat Shock Protein 90. Based on the Western-Blot principle, they are reserved for research laboratories.

7.2.2 Testing for circulating antigens

Various antigens can be tested in serum and other biological fluids (urine, cerebrospinal fluid, bronchoalveolar lavage fluid).

7.2.2.1 D-arabinitol

D-arabinitol, whether measured in urine or serum, has been shown to be an interesting marker of deep candidiasis [202]. It is a pentose produced by all *Candida* species except *C. glabrata* and *C. krusei*.

7.2.2.2 Mannans

Mannans represent the major antigens of *the Candida* wall. Three tests are currently on the market:

- Pastorex® Candida test (Bio-Rad)
- Platelia® Candida Ag kit (Bio-Rad)
- Serion ELISA antigen Candida® test (Virion/Serion)

In invasive candidiasis, mannan antigens may be positive several days before *Candida* isolation from a sterile site sample. However, this polysaccharide is only transiently found in serum. This means that regular serological monitoring of at-risk patients, with repeated sampling, is necessary, as mannan antigens are found transiently in the blood. The combined detection of anti-mannan antibodies and circulating mannans, combined with repeated sampling, is an approach that has demonstrated its value in terms of sensitivity and early diagnosis [203].

7.2.2.3 B (1,3) - D glucans

$\beta(1,3)$-D glucans are polysaccharides which, along with chitin, are major components of the *Candida* wall. In the heart of systemic candidiasis, they are detectable on average 10 days before the appearance of the first clinical signs.

The detection of $\beta(1,3)$-D glucans was included in the new EORTC (European organization for research and treatment of cancer) diagnostic criteria in 2008, but experience with these tests remains limited. To increase diagnostic sensitivity, some authors recommend combining the detection of these fungal markers with the detection of mannans, or even with molecular biology [204].

7.3 The benefits of molecular biology

Molecular biology techniques (PCR) can be used to diagnose, identify or type strains. Unlike the search for specific antibodies, the patient's immune status is not taken into account.

PCR enables DNA sequences to be amplified. What's more, it can theoretically be used for early diagnosis, replacing the need for blood cultures, with high sensitivity and specificity.

In recent years, real-time PCR techniques have experienced significant growth. They enable the simultaneous detection, quantitative and qualitative analysis of amplified DNA. Two systems widely used in bacteriology and virology, the TaqMan® (Perkin-Elmer, Applied Biosystems) and Lightcycler® (Roche Molecular Systems), currently enable this type of analysis [205].

The combination of a pair of universal primers and several pairs of specific primers or probes enables the simultaneous detection of several species in the same sample.

Nested PCR, whose performance is comparable to that of conventional PCR. Its principle is to first use a pair of "external" primers, and then use a pair of "internal" primers on this amplicon, often of small size. This avoids hybridization on a site other than the target, and therefore increases the specificity of the analysis, all the more so as the number of cycles is higher.

7.4 Diagnostic criteria of the European Organization for Research and Treatment of Cancers (EORTC) [166]

Classification of infectious episodes of systemic candidiasis is based in particular on the definitions revised in 2008 by the Europe Organization for Research and Treatment of Cancer / Invasive Fungal Infections Cooperative Group and the National Institute of Allergy and Infectious Diseases Mycoses Study Group (EORTC/MSG).

The EORTC Review Committee is revising definitions to standardize the inclusion of patients in clinical trials. Depending on their level of probability, invasive mycoses are classified as proven, probable or possible infections. As a general rule, infections are said to be proven when culture of a site deemed sterile reveals a micromycete, and clinical and/or imaging evidence supports this diagnosis. The distinction between probable and possible infections is made by the absence of mycological evidence (culture of an open site, presence of specific antibodies and antigens) in the case of possible infections. A host susceptibility factor and favorable clinical signs are required for the latter two forms. In clinical practice, however, this classification should not be used as an absolute and strict rule for making or excluding a diagnosis of invasive mycoses. Indeed, it has certain limitations, such as not taking into account the particularities of immunodepression or patients hospitalized in intensive care.

8 TREATMENT OF SYSTEMIC CANDIDIASIS

8.1 Introduction

The incidence of invasive candidiasis has risen sharply in recent years, especially among frail patients. This is due to a number of factors, such as the increasing use of immunosuppressive treatments in transplantation and autoimmune diseases, the use of aplasiant chemotherapy, and the multiplication of invasive procedures, which has necessitated an increase in the use of systemic antifungals to combat mortality, which remains high and worrying.

Antifungal therapy remains very costly, and to solve this problem we need to respect the proper use of this treatment and control its cost [206,207].

8.2 HISTORY

The first antifungal to be used was Griseofulvin, discovered in 1939, followed in 1951 by the Polyene family with Nystatin and Amphotericin. In 1957, 5-Fluorocytosine was discovered, and a year later the Azole class appeared, with Miconazole and Econazole. It was not until a quarter of a century later that new products appeared: ketoconazole (1983), the Triazole group with Fluconazole in 1990 and Itraconazole in 1993. Subsequently, new galenic forms of Amphotericin B were marketed: phospholipid complexes (1997) and liposomal forms (1998), improving renal tolerance and enabling higher doses of this active ingredient to be administered. In 2001, a new class of antifungal agents was added to the therapeutic arsenal: Echinocandins. Three molecules are currently available: Caspofungin, Anidulafungin and Micafungin [208]. In 2002, Voriconazole [209] was launched on the market, followed by Posaconazole [210] in 2006.

New triazoles, such as Ravuconazole and Isavuconazole, are now in the advanced stages of development.

8.3 STRUCTURE AND MECHANISMS OF ACTION

8.3.1 Amphotericin B

Amphotericin B is a fungicide derived from the cultivation of a fungus (Streptomyces nodosus), a soil actinomycete [211]. It is a complex molecule with 2 poles, one hydrophilic and the other hydrophobic.

Amphotericin B's mechanism of action involves dimerization of the molecule, enabling it to expose its hydrophobic poles. This dimer has a strong affinity for ergosterol, an essential component of the fungal membrane, enabling it to become embedded in this membrane. It thus forms channels releasing water and ions from the fungal cell, inducing its lysis (Figure 23).

A number of formulations are available: a deoxycholate formulation and 3 lipid formulations to limit toxicity and improve tolerance.

8.3.2 Nucleotide analogues

5 Fluorocytosine (5-FC) is a fluorinated pyrimidine converted to 5 Fluorouracil after penetration into the fungal cell by a fungal cytoplasmic enzyme, cytosine deaminase. Fluorouracil is then incorporated into RNA in place of uracil, thus altering the coding of fungal proteins (Figure 23). Its bioavailability and diffusion is excellent, including in cerebrospinal fluid.

8.3.3 Les Azolés

All Azoles have an identical mechanism of action. They inhibit the CYTP450-dependent enzyme lanosterol 14α-demethylase, which catalyzes an essential step in the biosynthesis of ergosterol from lanosterol, a compound essential for maintaining the integrity of the fungal membrane. This enzyme is not present in humans, which explains the specificity of Azoles for the fungal membrane (Figure 23).

8.3.4 Caspofungin

Caspofungin is a lipopeptide of the Echinocandin family, derived from the fermentation of a fungus: Glarea lozoyensis. It inhibits the synthesis of β (1,3) D-glucan in the cell wall of fungi such as *Candida* and Aspergillus. Inhibition of the B (1,3) D-glucan synthetase enzyme therefore represents a distinct mechanism of action from other antifungals (polyenes and azoles), as it is located in the fungal cell wall and not on the fungal membrane. This different mode of action will pave the way for combination antifungal treatments, as the spectra of action of antifungal agents frequently overlap, as we shall see below (Figure 23).

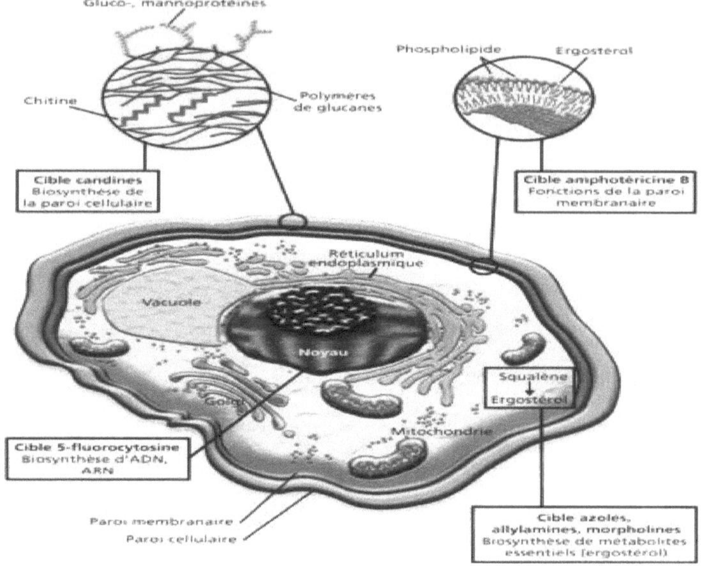

Figure. 23: Cellular targets of the antifungal families [7].

8.4 SPECTRUM OF ACTION

The in vitro sensitivities of the main antifungal agents against the main *Candida* species are listed in Table III [212].

As we have said, contemporary antifungal agents target the fungal wall or membrane. This action should therefore be aspecific. However, the spectrum of antifungal agents varies according to family, from broad to more restricted.

Amphotericin B is a powerful, broad-spectrum antifungal agent, including zygomycetes, and remains the systemic antifungal of choice. Its main drawback is its renal toxicity, especially in the deoxycholate form. Lipid formulations of this molecule, AmB liposamale (Ambisome®) and AmB lipidique (Abelcet®), have been developed to reduce this nephrotoxicity, and are better tolerated.

Table. III: Spectra of antifungal agents

	AmB	Fluco	Itraco	Vorico	Posaco	Caspo
C albicans	S	S	S	S	NE	S
C glabrata	S/I	SDD/R	SDD/R	S/ ?	NE	S
Cparapsilosis	S	S	S	S	NE	S/ ?
C tropicalis	S	SDD/S	S	S	NE	S
C krusei	S/I	R	SDD/RS	S	NE	S
C luisitaniae	S/R	S	S	S	NE	S
A fumigatus	S	R	S/R	S	S	S/R
A flavus	S	R	S	S	S	S
A terreus	S	R	S	S	S	SR

[Hochart S et al. Systemic antifungals: Part 1: pharmaceutical elements. Le Pharmacien Hospitalier . Volume 43, Issue 173, June 2008, Pages 103-109]

S: sensitive, **I:** intermediate, **R:** resistant, **SDD:** dose-dependent sensitivity, **S/?** Some cases of resistance have been described, **S/R:** variable sensitivity depending on species or strain, **NE:** not evaluated.

Flucytocin (5-FC): fungistatic, active on most *Candida. However,* 30% of *C tropicalis and C krusei* strains are resistant.

Fluconazole, the first of the triazoles, includes *C. albicans, C. tropicalis* and *C. parapsilosis* in its spectrum. It is not very active on *C. glabrata*, and doses of 800 mg are often required to treat this species.

Fluconazole is inactive on *C. krusei*. Some strains of *C. albicans* are resistant to fluconazole.

Itraconazole (Sporanox®) has an antifungal spectrum similar to fluconazole against *Candida* species.

Voriconazole (Vfend®) is the first of a new generation of triazole derivatives. It is intrinsically more active than Fluconazole against *Candida* strains, with MICs 4 to 16 times lower, and is active against *Candida glabrata* and *Candida krusei*. Its use in prophylaxis has recently led to the emergence of serious infections with these fungi in immunocompromised patients [213].

Posaconazole (Noxafil®), the latest Triazole to be marketed, has an as yet ill-defined spectrum with regard to the *Candida* genus.

Caspofungin is an Echinocandin with fungicidal activity against a wide variety of pathogens, including *Candida* species. It is active against *Candida albicans* varieties sensitive or resistant to Fluconazole. However, it is less active than Amphotericin B against strains of *C. parapsilosis* [214].

8.5 GALENIC FORMS AND MARKETED DOSAGES

8.5.1 Amphotericin B

Amphotericin is marketed in three different dosage forms (Tab. 4):

- A micellar solution using deoxycholate (Fungizone®) for oral, intravenous and respiratory use.
- A lamellar lipid complex (Abelcet®) for intravenous use only
- Inclusion in a liposome (Ambisome®) composed of phosphatidylcholine, distearoyl, phosphatidylglycerol and cholesterol for intravenous administration.

The attenuation of Amphotericin B's lipophilic character, achieved by association with lipid structures, is intended to improve its tolerability, and in particular to reduce the frequency of induction of renal disorders. The stability of these vectorized forms also seems to be linked to less accumulation in the distal renal tubules [215].

8.5.2 Les Azolés

Azoles are available in dry oral form, as a solution or oral suspension, and as an injectable solution. The forms and strengths available on the market are shown in Table IV.

8.5.3 Caspofungin

Caspofungin is only available as an injectable solution (Table IV). Its very bulky structure prevents enteral absorption.

Table IV: Marketed forms and dosages of systemic antifungals

	Speciality	Dry oral form	Liquid oral form	Injectable form	External shape
Ampho B	Fungizone®	250 mg capsules	10% suspension	50 mg powder	3% lotion
	Abelcet®			Susp 5 mg/ml (20 ml)	
	Ambisome®			50 mg powder	
Fluconazole	Triflucan® and generics	Capsules 50,100 and 200 mg	Powder for oral suspension : 50 and 200 mg/5 ml	2 mg/ml solution in 50, 100 and 200 ml	
Itraconazole	Sporanox®	100mg capsules	Oral solution 10 mg/ml	Solution containing 250 mg.	
Voriconazole	Vfend®	50 % tablet and 200 mg	40 mg/ml oral suspension	Powder for IV solution 200 mg	
Posaconazole	Noxafil®		40 mg/ml oral suspension		
Caspofungin	Cancidas®			Powder for perfm50 and 70 mg.	

[Hochart S et al. Systemic antifungals: Part 1: pharmaceutical elements. Le Pharmacien Hospitalier . Volume 43, Issue 173, June 2008, Pages 103-109]

8.6 Therapeutic choice criteria

Different possible therapeutic strategies based on the stage of diagnosis have been described, such as prophylactic, empirical, preventive and targeted antifungal therapy.

Prophylactic treatment refers to the preventive administration of an antifungal agent to patients at risk of CS without attributable signs and symptoms. Empirical therapy is defined as the initiation of antifungal treatment in patients at high risk of CS with established clinical signs and symptoms, but without microbiological documentation, while preventive therapy is applied when the treatment decision is based on an early diagnostic test. Finally, targeted therapy requires identification of the pathogen to be defined.

8.6.1 Targeted antifungal treatment (curative) [216]

[Update from IDSA (Infectious Dsease Society of America 2016].

8.6.1.1 Treatment of CS in non-neutropenic patients e

1. Echinocandin (aspofungin: 70 mg loading dose, then 50 mg daily; Micafungin: 100 mg daily; Anidulafungin: 200 mg loading dose, then 100 mg daily) is recommended as initial therapy.

2. Fluconazole, intravenous or oral, 800 mg (12 mg / kg) loading dose then 400 mg (6 mg / kg) daily is an acceptable alternative to an Echinocandin as selected initial therapy for patients who are not critically ill and who are considered unlikely to have a *Candida* species resistant to Fluconazole (strong recommendation, high-quality evidence).

3. Transition from Echinocandin to Fluconazole (usually within 5-7 days) is recommended for patients who are clinically stable, have isolates sensitive to Fluconazole (e.g. *C. albicans*), and have negative repeat blood cultures after initiation of antifungal therapy.

4. For infection due to *C. glabrata*, transition to a higher dose of Fluconazole 800 mg (12 mg / kg) daily or Voriconazole 200-300 mg (3-4 mg / kg) twice daily should only be considered in patients with Fluconazole or Voriconazole

sensitivity.

5. Lipid formulation Amphotericin B (AmB) (3-5 mg / kg per day) is a reasonable alternative in cases of intolerance, limited availability or resistance to other antifungal agents.

6. Transition from AmB to Fluconazole is recommended after 5-7 days in patients with Fluconazole-susceptible isolates, who are clinically stable and in whom repeat cultures on antifungal therapy are negative.

7. For patients suspected of being resistant to Azoles and Echinocandin, the lipid formulation AmB (3-5 mg / kg per day) is recommended.

8. Voriconazole 400 mg (6 mg / kg) twice daily, then 200 mg (3 mg / kg) twice daily is effective for candidemia, but offers little advantage over Fluconazole. It is recommended as oral therapy for certain cases of candidemia due to *C. krusei*.

9. All non-neutropenic patients with candidemia should have a dilated ophthalmological examination, preferably by an ophthalmologist, within the first week of diagnosis.

10. Blood cultures should be taken every day until candidemia disappears.

11. The recommended duration of treatment for candidiasis without obvious metastatic complications is 2 weeks after the last negative blood cultures and resolution of symptoms attributable to candidemia.

12. Central venous catheters (CVCs) should be removed as early as possible in the course of candidemia when the source is presumed to be the CVC. This decision should be individualized for each patient.

8.6.1.2 Treatment of CS in neutropenic patients

1. Echinocandin (Caspofungin: 70 mg loading dose, then 50 mg daily; Micafungin: 100 mg daily; Anidulafungin: 200 mg loading dose, then 100 mg daily) is recommended as initial therapy.

2. Lipid formula AmB, 3-5 mg / kg per day, is effective but a less attractive alternative due to the potential for toxicity.

3. Fluconazole, a loading dose of 800 mg (12 mg / kg), then 400 mg (6 mg / kg) per day, is an alternative for patients who are not seriously ill and have had no previous exposure to azoles.

4. Fluconazole, 400 mg (6 mg / kg) daily, can be used as a secondary treatment for patients with persistent neutropenia with clinical stability and presenting susceptible isolates and negative blood cultures.

5. Voriconazole, 400 mg (6 mg / kg) twice daily, then 200-300 mg (3-4 mg / kg) twice daily, can be used in situations where additional mold coverage is desired. Voriconazole can be used as a secondary treatment for clinically stable, neutropenic patients with negative blood cultures and isolates sensitive to voriconazole.

6. For infections due to *C. krusei*, an Echinocandin, a lipid formulation of AmB or Voriconazole is recommended.

7. Minimum recommended duration of treatment for candidemia without metastatic complications is 2 weeks after the last negative blood cultures and resolution of neutropenia and symptoms attributable to candidemia.

8. Choroidal and vitreous ophthalmological infections are minimal Dilated funduscopy should be performed within The first week after normalization of neutropenia.

9. In neutropenic patients, sources of candidiasis other than a CVC (e.g. gastrointestinal tract) must be considered on an individual basis.

10. Granulocyte transfusions may be considered in cases of persistent candidemia with anticipated prolonged neutropenia.

8.6.1.3 Treatment of chronic disseminated candidiasis (hepatosplenic)

1. Initial therapy with lipid formulation AmB, 3-5 mg / kg per day or an Echinocandin (Micafungin: 100 mg per day, Caspofungin: 70 mg loading dose, then 50 mg per day; Or Anidulafungin: 200 mg loading dose, then 100 mg per day), for several weeks is recommended, followed by oral Fluconazole, 400 mg (6 mg / kg) daily, for patients who are unlikely to have fluconazole resistance.

2. Therapy should continue until lesions resolve. Premature discontinuation of antifungal therapy may lead to relapse.

3. If chemotherapy or hematopoietic cell transplantation is required, it should not be delayed due to the presence of chronic disseminated candidiasis, and antifungal therapy should be continued throughout the high-risk period to

prevent relapse.

4. For patients with debilitating persistent fevers, short-term treatment (1-2 weeks) with non-steroidal anti-inflammatory drugs or corticosteroids may be considered.

8.6.1.4 Isolation of *Candida* species from the respiratory tract and antifungal therapy

Candida growth from respiratory secretions usually indicates colonization and rarely requires antifungal treatment (strong recommendation, moderate quality evidence).

8.6.1.5 Treatment of *Candida* endocarditis

1. For native valvular endocarditis, lipid formulation AmB, 3-5 mg / kg daily, with or without Flucytosine, 25 mg / kg 4 times daily, or a high-dose Echinocandin (Caspofungin 150 mg daily, Micafungin 150 mg daily or Anidulafungin 200 mg daily) is recommended for initial therapy.

2. Staged treatment with Fluconazole, 400-800 mg (6-12 mg /Kg) per day, is recommended for patients with susceptible *candida* isolates, have demonstrated clinical stability and have eliminated *Candida* from the bloodstream.

3. Oral Voriconazole, 200-300 mg (3-4 mg / kg) twice daily, or Posaconazole tablets, 300 mg daily, can be used as therapy for isolates that are sensitive to these agents but not to Fluconazole.

4. Valve replacement is recommended; treatment should continue for at least 6 weeks after surgery, and for longer in patients with perivalvular abscesses and other complications.

5. For patients unable to undergo valve replacement, Fluconazole, 400-800 mg (6-12 mg /Kg) daily, if isolate susceptible, is recommended.

6. For valve prosthesis endocarditis, the same antifungal regimens suggested for native valve endocarditis are recommended. Chronic prophylactic antifungal treatment with Fluconazole, 400-800 mg (6-12 mg / kg) daily, is recommended to prevent relapse (strong recommendation, low-quality evidence).

8.6.1.6 Treatment for osteoarticular *Candida* infections

- #### *Candida* osteomyelitis

1. Fluconazole, 400 mg (6 mg / kg) per day, for 6-12 months or an Echinocandin (Caspofungin 50-70 mg per day, Micafungin 100 mg per day, or Anidulafungin 100 mg per day) for at least 2 weeks followed by Fluconazole, 400 mg (6 mg / kg) per day, for 6-12 months is recommended.
2. Lipid formulation AmB, 3-5 mg / kg per day, for at least 2 weeks followed by Fluconazole, 400 mg (6 mg / kg) per day, for 6 to 12 months is a less attractive alternative.
3. Surgical debridement is recommended in certain cases.

- #### *Candida* septic arthritis

1. Fluconazole, 400 mg (6 mg / kg) daily, for 6 weeks or an Echinocandin (Caspofungin 50-70 mg daily, Micafungin 100 mg daily, or Anidulafungin 100 mg daily) for 2 weeks followed by Fluconazole, 400 mg (6 mg / kg) daily, for at least 4 weeks is recommended.
2. Lipid formula AmB, 3-5 mg / kg per day, for 2 weeks, followed by Fluconazole, 400 mg (6 mg / kg) per day, for at least 4 weeks is a less attractive alternative.
3. Surgical drainage is indicated in all cases of septic arthritis (Strong recommendation, moderate quality evidence).
4. For septic arthritis involving a prosthesis, removal of a device is recommended.
5. If the prosthesis cannot be removed, chronic suppression with Fluconazole, 400 mg (6 mg / kg) per day, if the isolate is susceptible, is recommended.

8.6.1.7 Treatment of *Candida* endophthalmitis

1. For isolates sensitive to Fluconazole / Voriconazole, Fluconazole loading dose 800 mg (12 mg / kg), then 400-800 mg (6-12 mg / kg) daily or Voriconazole loading dose 400 mg (6 mg / kg) intravenously twice daily, then 300 mg (4 mg / kg) intravenously or orally twice daily is recommended.
2. For isolates resistant to Fluconazole / Voriconazole, AmB liposomes, 3-5 mg / kg intravenously daily, with or without oral Flucytosine, 25 mg / kg 4 times daily is recommended.
3. With macular involvement, the antifungal agents mentioned above, plus

intravitreal injection of AmB deoxycholate, 5-10 μg / 0.1 ml sterile water, or Voriconazole, 100 μg /0.1 ml sterile water or normal saline, to ensure a high level of antifungal activity is recommended.

4. Treatment duration should be at least 4-6 weeks, with the final duration depending on lesion resolution.

8.6.1.8 Treatment for urinary tract infections caused by *Candida*

- **Symptomatic *Candida* cystitis**

1. For organisms sensitive to Fluconazole, oral Fluconazole 200 mg (3 mg / kg) daily for 2 weeks.

2. For Fluconazole-resistant *C. glabrata*, AmB deoxycholate, 0.3-0.6 mg / kg daily for 1 to 7 days. Oral FLucytosine, 25 mg / kg 4 times a day for 7 to 10 days is recommended.

3. For *C. krusei*, AmB deoxycholate, 0.3-0.6 mg / kg per day, for 1-7 days is recommended.

4. Elimination of an indwelling bladder catheter, if possible, is strongly recommended.

5. Irrigation of the bladder with AmB deoxycholate, 50 mg/day for 5 days, can be useful in treating cystitis due to Fluconazole-resistant species such as *C. glabrata* and *C. krusei*.

- **Treatment of *Candida* pyelonephritis**

1. For organisms sensitive to Fluconazole, oral Fluconazole, 200-400 mg (3-6 mg / kg) per day for 2 weeks is recommended.

2. For Fluconazole-resistant *C. glabrata*, AmB deoxycholate, 0.3-0.6 mg / kg daily for 1 to 7 days with or without oral Flucytosine, 25 mg / kg 4 times daily, is recommended.

3. For Fluconazole-resistant *C. glabrata*, monotherapy with oral Flucytosine, 25 mg / kg 4 times daily for 2 weeks.

4. For *C. krusei*, AmB deoxycholate, 0.3-0.6 mg / kg per day, for 1-7 days is recommended.

5. Elimination of urinary tract obstruction is strongly recommended (strong recommendation, poor quality evidence).

8.6.1.9 Treatment of central nervous system infections

Treatment is based on liposomal AmB, possibly combined with Flucytosine for 10 weeks. It is important to note that Echinocandins are not indicated in this context.

Finally, in the case of internal ventricular bypass, removal of the material (with placement of an external ventricular bypass if necessary) is recommended [171].

8.6.2 Empirical antifungal treatment

Early identification of risk factors for the development of CS, such as peritonitis, abdominal surgery, previous administration of broad-spectrum antibiotics, parenteral nutrition, central catheters, previous colonization with *Candida spp* ,and mechanical ventilation [110,121,217], have become the cornerstone of empirical treatment of fungal infections in the ICU in order to reduce the high mortality associated with these infections [218,219]. In a multicenter retrospective setting, Ostrosky-Zeichner and colleagues (2007) [220] created a prediction rule for CS. The rule was obtained by analyzing a group of 2,890 patients, whose incidence of CS was 3% (88 cases). Statistical modeling revealed a particularly high risk for patients undergoing systemic antibiotic treatment (days 1-3) or with an indwelling central venous catheter (days 1-3) and at least two of the following factors: total parenteral nutrition (days 1-3), any dialysis (days 1-3), any major surgery, pancreatitis, any use of steroids, or use of other immunosuppressive agents. The rule was associated with a sensitivity of 34%, a specificity of 90% and a PPV and NPV of 1% and 97%, respectively. This rule applies to around 10% of patients who remain in the unit for > 4 days, and around 10% of patients to whom this rule is applied will develop proven or probable CS. In this study, patients with a combination of diabetes mellitus, hemodialysis, use of total parenteral nutrition or receipt of broad-spectrum antibiotics had a CS rate of 16.6%. This compared with a rate of 5.1% in patients who did not have these characteristics (P = 0.001). 52% of patients who remained in the ICU for ≥ 4 days complied with this rule, and the rule captured 78% of patients who ultimately developed CS.

Candida score: a Spanish group has reported on the development of a bedside scoring system that enables early antifungal treatment of suspected candidemia in non-neuropenic ICU patients [221]. This "*Candida* score" is based on the predictive value of previously reported risk factors. The authors found that several factors were independently associated with a greater risk of proven candidiasis infection. Scores for individual factors were: parenteral nutrition (+0.908), previous surgery (+0.997), multifocal *Candida* colonization (+1.112) and severe sepsis (+2.038). The authors concluded that a "*Candida* score" > 2.5 could accurately select patients who would benefit from early antifungal treatment (sensitivity 81%, specificity 74%).

8.6.3 Preventive antifungal treatment

Poor results are partly associated with difficulties in establishing the diagnosis at an early stage of infection. Blood culture results are positive in only 50% of invasive *Candida* infections. Positive cultures of samples from non-sterile body sites may be related to colonization or infection, and it can be difficult to distinguish between them. Non-culture-based diagnostic tests can provide a useful complement to these more traditional approaches. Corrected colonization index : Piarroux and colleagues (2004) [222] evaluated the efficacy of preventive antifungal therapy in preventing proven candidiasis in critically ill surgical patients, using a corrected colonization index (CCI) (ratio of highly positive samples to the total number of samples cultured) to measure the intensity of mucosal colonization by *Candida spp.* Patients with an ICC value ≥0.4 received early preventive antifungal treatment with fluconazole, and the incidence of proven candidiasis acquired in intensive care decreased significantly from 2.2 to 0%.

8.6.4 Prophylactic antifungal treatment

The implementation of targeted antifungal prophylaxis has proved effective in some ICUs [223]. The results of randomized controlled trials [78, 100,224] support the efficacy of Azole prophylaxis in high-risk, non-neutropenic ICU patients, reducing the incidence of *Candida* infection but not mortality. Three recently published meta-analyses have attempted to assess the impact of Fluconazole prophylaxis on the incidence of fungal infections and mortality in critically ill surgical patients [225, 226,227]. The meta-analysis by Shorr and colleagues [226] demonstrated that prophylactic administration of Fluconazole in intensive care patients appears to successfully reduce the rate of mycoses, but this strategy does not improve survival. The second meta-analysis by Cruciani and colleagues (2005) [225] showed that patients who received azole prophylaxis (Fluconazole and ketoconazole) experienced an 80% relative risk reduction in candidemia, 31.5% relative risk reduction in overall mortality and 79.4% in mortality attributable *to Candida* infections. Finally, Playford and colleagues (2006) [227] reported a reduction in IC incidence of around 50% and overall mortality of around 25%. Patient subgroups that may benefit most from IC prophylaxis may include patients with upper gastrointestinal perforation [100,224], patients with abundant *Candida* colonization [222] and patients with severe acute pancreatitis [228].

PRACTICAL STUDY

9 TYPE, SCOPE AND PERIOD OF STUDY

This is a prospective, descriptive, bicentric study carried out in the BATNA University Hospital and Anti-Cancer Center. The study was conducted over a three-year period (January 1, 2016 to December 31, 2018).

10 PATIENT RECRUITMENT

Our study covered all patients, of both sexes, hospitalized at BATNA CHU and CAC during the above-mentioned study period, whatever the department and reason for hospitalization, aged≥ 16 years, having undergone at least one deep sampling from a normally sterile site (blood, cerebrospinal fluid, peritoneal fluid, joint puncture fluid, etc.), sent to our Parasitology-Mycology department for mycological analysis.

10.1 Inclusion criteria:

- Our study included all patients with at least one *Candida spp-positive* deep-seated swab in direct examination and/or culture.
- Each *Candida-positive* deep swab is considered a proven case of systemic Candidiasis according to EORTC (2008) diagnostic criteria.

10.2 Exclusion criteria

The following were excluded from our study:

- Patients hospitalized in the neonatology or pediatrics departments.
- Patients with deep smears positive for yeasts other than *Candida.*
- Patients with negative deep samples.
- Patients undergoing prophylactic antifungal treatment.

10.3 Data sheet

An information sheet was drawn up for each patient included in our study (with proven CS) [Appendix1].

Data were collected on :

- Patient demographics.
- Mycological data.
- Clinical data
- Therapeutic data.
- Patient progress.

10.4 Sample size

To estimate the required sample size, we used the following formula:

$$n = [z_\alpha^2 * p(1-p)] / i^2$$

- n: Minimum sample size required to obtain significant results for a given event and risk level.
- z_α : Confidence level (the typical value for the 95% confidence level is 1.96)
- p: Estimated proportion of population with the characteristic (p=10%).
- i : Margin of error (accuracy) = 0.05

$$n = (1.96)^2 \times 0.10 \times (1-0.10)/(0.05)^2 = 138.29 \text{ so } n=138$$

So the minimum sample size to be representative with a 95% confidence level is 138.

In our study, our sample size is 157, so it is representative.

11 MATERIALS AND METHODS S

11.1   Laboratory equipment

- **Reagents and solutions**
    1. Cotton blue.
    2. Sterile physiological water.
    3. Ready-to-use suspension media for the Api Candida gallery (Biomerieux) (Appendix2).
    4. Reagents and solutions from Bio-rad's PLATELIA® Candida Ag Plus Kit (see Appendix 3).
    5. PLATELIA® Candida Ab Plus Kit reagents and solutions (see Appendix 4).

- **Laboratory equipment and consumables**
    1. Graduated cylinder (500 ml).
    2. Sample dilution tubes.
    3. 3 ml Eppendorf tubes.
    4. Micropipettes: 10 µl, 100 µl, 200 µl.
    5. Yellow and blue tips.
    6. Petri dishes.

- **Culture media**
    1. Sabouraud-Chloramphenicol media in 10 cc tubes.
    2. Sabouraud-Chloramphenicol - Actidione media in 10 cc tubes.
    3. CHROMagar Candida media in 180 cc bottle.
    4. Rice cream media in 10 cc tubes.

- **Equipment**
    1. Optical microscope.
    2. Centrifuge at 5000 and 10000 rpm.
    3. Bain marie set to 100°C.
    4. Vortex.
    5. Automate (ELISA microplate reader).
    6. Refrigerator for storage of serum samples and reagents to be used (2 - 8 °C).

7. Incubation ovens set at 27 °C and 37°C.

11.2 Diagnostic approach to systemic candidiasis in the Parasitology-Mycology laboratory at BATNA University Hospital

11.2.1 Samples

All patients with suspected systemic candidiasis received one or more deep swabs, depending on the patient's clinical context.

Our task was to carry out the mycological examination and select *Candida-positive* samples for inclusion in our study.

A distinction is made between :

➤ **Blood cultures** (Figure 24)

During the study period, we received blood samples taken at the time of fever peak, inoculated in nutrient broth medium and sent to our laboratory for mycological study. Blood culture bottles were incubated at 37°C for 24 hours. These broths are reseeded on specific mycological media (Sabouraud -Chloramphenicol with and without Actidione). Incubation lasts 2-5 days.

For each patient, a blood volume of 10 ml is recommended.

A negative blood culture does not rule out the diagnosis of candidemia; however, a single positive blood culture confirms the diagnosis.

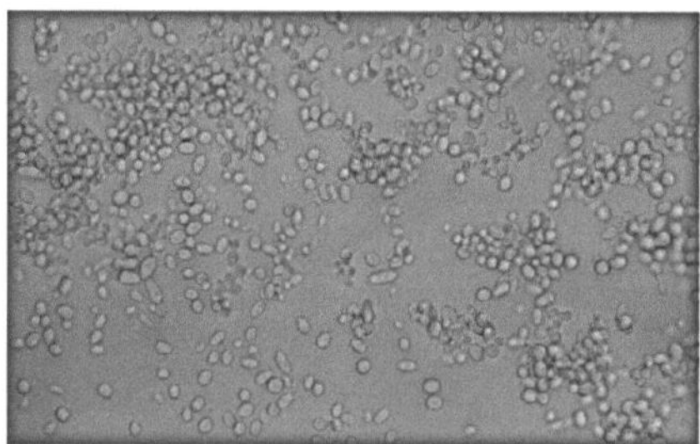

Figure. 24. Direct microscopic examination of a blood culture positive for *Candida*

➢ Other sampling :

- Cerebrospinal fluid (CSF).
- Peritoneal fluid.
- Joint puncture fluid.
- Biopsies (valvular vegetations).

The other samples mentioned above are inoculated directly into Sabouraud-Chloramphenicol ±Actidone medium for 24-48 hours at 37°C.

All patients with at least one deep swab positive for *Candida spp*, i.e. with proven CS, were systematically given 05 superficial swabs (buccal, rectal or stool, urine, nasal and ear) using sterile swabs, in order to calculate the Pittet colonization index. These superficial swabs were taken in collaboration with the attending physicians.

Samples are sent immediately to the Parasitology-Mycology laboratory at BATNA University Hospital.

All samples, whether deep or superficial, are examined directly and cultured.

11.2.2 Direct examination

Between slide and coverslip, with or without cotton blue, to detect budding yeasts with or without pseudofilaments.

11.2.3 Cultivation

Samples are inoculated by isolating and progressively depleting the inoculum on the agar (by quadrant, star or rotation).

Swabs are unloaded directly.

After homogenization, urine is inoculated onto agar plates.

Each sample was seeded on two media (Sabouraud-Chloramphenicol with and without Actidionne).

Incubation takes place at 37°C for 48 hours, and up to 5 days for blood cultures.

Macroscopic examination of positive cultures shows white, moist colonies with a smooth, shiny surface (Figure 25).

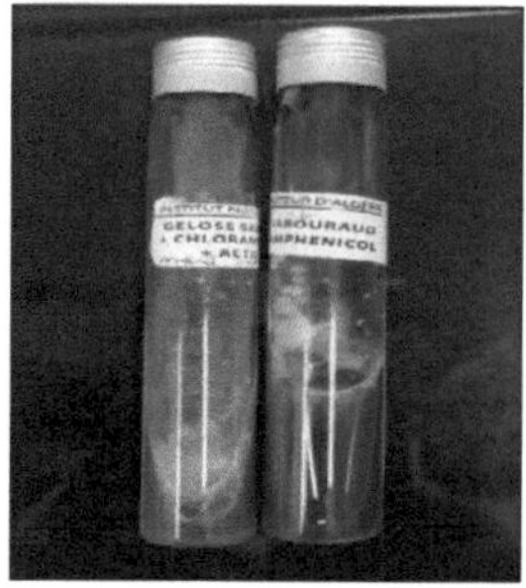

Figure. 25: Positive blood cultures on both Sabouraud Chloramphenicol and Sabouraud Chloramphenicol - Actidione media.

11.2.4   Identification

11.2.4.1   Identification of *Candida albicans* species

Based on two tests:

Blastesis (or Filamentation) test: performed by incubating the isolate for 3 to 4 hours in serum at 37°C. *Candida albicans* is then identified by the production of a thin germ tube of homogeneous diameter with no constriction at its base, emerging from the mother cell (Figure 26).

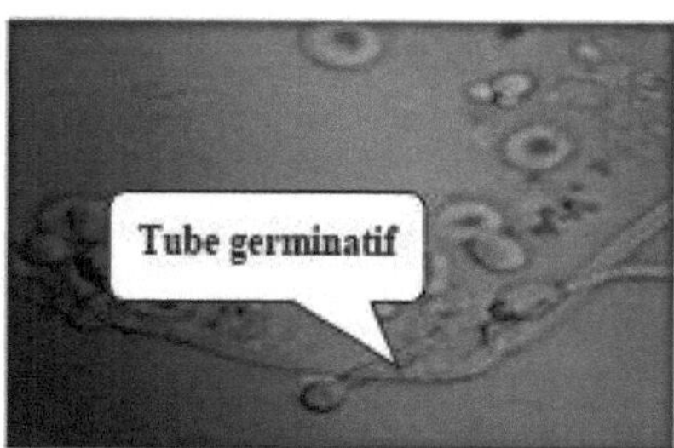

Figure. 26: Positive filamentation test

Chlamydosporulation test: based on a 24 to 48-hour culture at 27°C of the isolate in deep streaks in Rice cream medium. *Candida albicans* is identified by the production of chlamydospores (Figure 27).

86

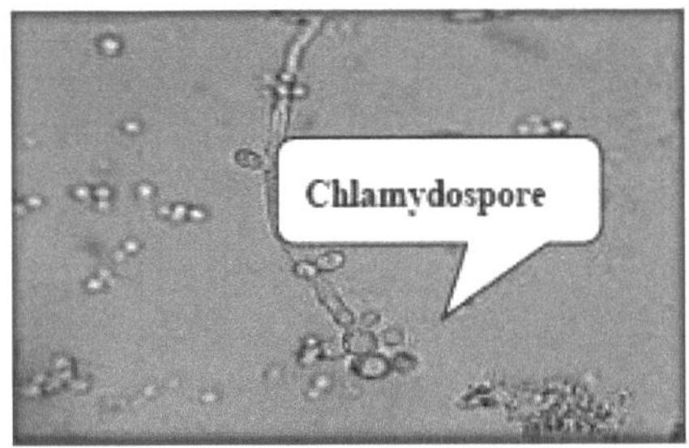

Figure. 27: Positive chlamydosporulation test

11.2.4.2   Identification of other species

Other *Candida* species were identified from cultures of deep samples (blood cultures, peritoneal fluid, cerebrospinal fluid, joint fluid) using the **API Candida** gallery **(BioMérieux)** see (Appendix 2).

The identification of *Candida* species from positive cultures of superficial samples was carried out by reseeding on selective **CHROMagar Candida** medium. This is a medium to which chromogenic substances are added, giving the colonies that develop there a particular coloration, which varies according to the species. In most cases, this coloration is based on the detection of hexosaminidase-type enzymatic activity (N-acetyl-α-D-galactosaminidase). Incubation takes place at 37°C for 48 hours. Colony color differs according to species (Figure 28).

C. albicans colonies are in green.

C. tropicalis colonies are shown in metallic blue.

C. krusei colonies are pale pink.

C parapsilosis colonies are cream-colored.

C glabrata colonies are in mauve.

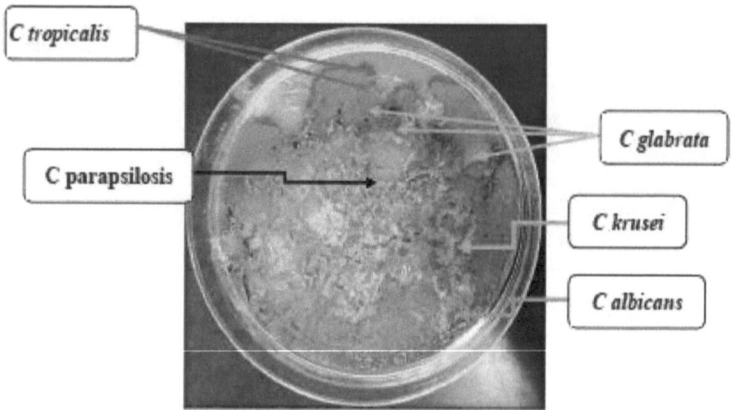

Figure. 28: Colony appearance on CHROMagar Candida medium

11.2.5 Calculating the colonization index

The colonization index is calculated as presented by Pittet: ratio between the number of positive sites and the total number of sites sampled [90].

Colonized patients: Patients with at least one positive peripheral site sample.

Non-colonized patients: These are patients with no positive peripheral site samples.

11.2.6 Determination of mannan antigenemia and mannan antibodies

Diagnosis of deep-rooted *Candida* infections remains difficult, given the non-specificity of clinical and biological signs, as well as blood cultures, which are positive late in 40% of cases. To remedy this diagnostic shortcoming, an ELISA assay for mannan antigen was performed using the PLATELIA® Candida Ag Plus Kit (Bio-rad) (see appendix 3), and an ELISA assay for polyclonal mannan antibodies was performed using the PLATELIA® Candida Ab Plus Kit (see appendix 4), on patient sera collected in a dry tube.

For each technique we calculated :

Sensitivity: is defined by the proportion of patients who have the disease of interest and whose test is positive.

Specificity: is defined by the proportion of patients who do not have the disease tested for and whose test is negative.

11.2.7 Statistical analysis of data

The first step was to carry out a descriptive analysis of the population (prevalence, demographic, clinical, biological and prognostic analysis).

Categorical variables are expressed in figures and percentages.

For quantitative variables, we calculated the mean and standard deviation.

Data entry and graphical and tabular representations were made using Microsoft Excel 2007.

Statistical analyses were carried out using the **BiostaTG** website.

Uni- and multivariate analyses were performed using the Chi2 test. For each statistical test used, the test was considered significant when **P** (significance level) was < **0.05**.

Determination of the sensitivity and specificity of immunological techniques was carried out using the website: **www. aly-abbara.com**

11.3 Ethical aspects

Ethical rules relating to medical confidentiality were followed. Anonymity is guaranteed, and patient characteristics are analyzed without recording the patient's name or geographical coordinates.

Informed consent must be obtained before the patient is included in the study.

The study was carried out entirely in the open, **and** for each requesting department, we obtained authorization from the head physician to access patients' medical records and collect the various data.

Biological test results were communicated to the attending physicians.

12 RESULTS

During the study period (between   January 1^{ier} 2016 and December 31 2018), 157 patients underwent at least one sampling from a normally sterile deep site (Blood, CSF,

Peritoneal fluid, Joint puncture fluid...), sent to the Parasitology -Mycology laboratory at BATNA University Hospital. We performed a direct examination and culture for each deep sample, and retained all samples that tested positive for *Candida* (in direct examination and/or culture).

12.1 Global data

- **Overall patient distribution**

We report in (Figure 29) the overall distribution of patients who had undergone at least one deep sampling sent to our laboratory for mycological study.

Out of 157 patients :

- A total of 91 patients (57.96%) had negative deep smears (PPN) for *Candida spp*, and were therefore excluded from our study.
- A total of 66 patients had at least one positive deep swab (PPP) for *Candida spp*, of whom 3 patients (1.91%) were hospitalized on the neonatal ward. Thus excluded from our study.
- Thus, a total of 63 patients (40.13%) were included in our study.

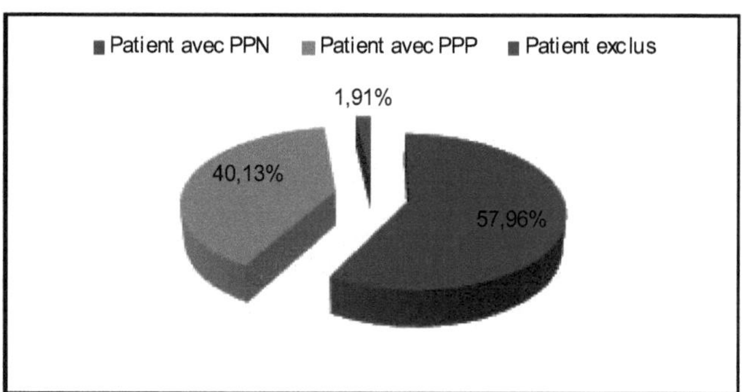

Figure. 29: Overall patient distribution.

(**PPN**: negative deep sampling, **PPP**: positive deep sampling)

- **Overall distribution of *Candida* spp-positive deep samples**

Table V shows the overall distribution of deep samples positive for *Candida spp*.

Table. V: Overall distribution of *Candida spp-positive* deep samples

Type of sampling	Number	Frequency
Blood culture	59	85,5%
Peritoneal fluids	5	7,25%
Cerebrospinal fluid	3	4,35 %
Joint puncture fluid	1	1,45%
Valvular vegetation	1	1,45%
Total	69	100%

- **Overall distribution of diagnosed cases of systemic candidiasis.**

Each *Candida spp-positive* sample received corresponds to a proven case of systemic candidiasis according to the **EORTC** 2008 classification criteria.

Table VI shows the overall distribution of diagnosed cases of systemic candidiasis.

Table. VI: Overall distribution of diagnosed CS cases

Type of CS	Number	Frequency
Candidemie	59	85,50%
Peritonitis	5	7,25%
Endocarditis	1	1,45%
Arthritis	1	1,45%
Meningitis	3	4,35%
Total	69	100%

Each patient included in our study underwent 05 peripheral swabs (urine, stool, buccal, nasal and ear) to calculate the Pittet colonization index. A total of 315 peripheral swabs were taken.

12.2 Demographics

Figure 30 shows the distribution of patients by age.

The mean age of patients in our study was 48.31 years, extremes (16 and 83 years), median = 48 years, standard deviation =18.5.

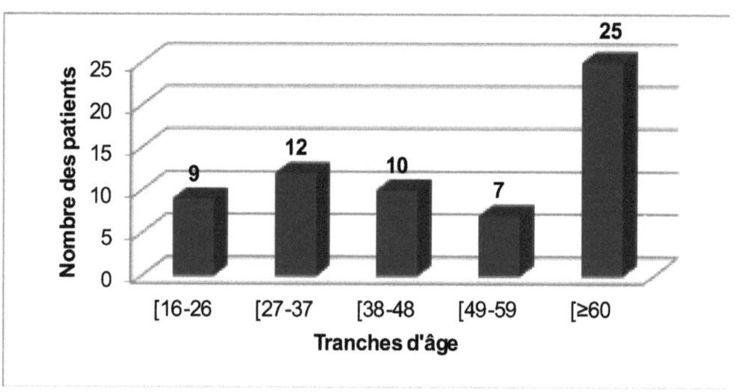

Figure. 30: patient age distribution

Figure 31 shows the distribution of patients by gender.

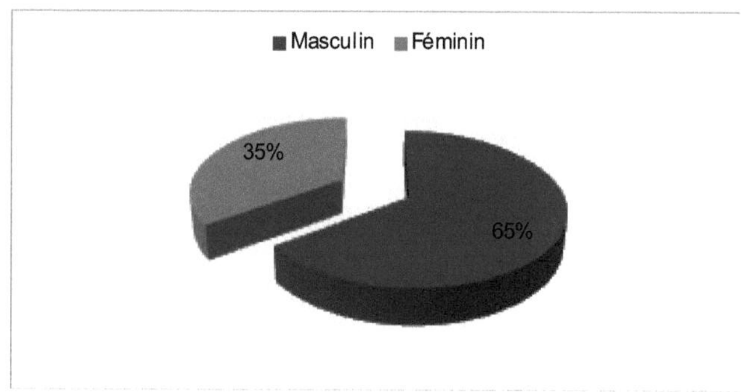

Fig. 31: Distribution of patients by sex

Of the 63 patients, 41 were male (65%) and 22 female (35%).

The sex ratio favored male patients with (M/F) = 1.86.

12.3 Hospitalization services

Table VII shows the distribution of patients by hospital ward.

Table. VII: Distribution of CS cases by hospital ward

Hospitalization department	Workforce	Percentage
Medical resuscitation (REAM)	28	40,6%
Surgical resuscitation (REAC)	4	5,8%
Internal medicine	3	4,35%

Nephrology	10	14,5%
Hematology	9	13,04
Cancer Center (CAC)	9	13,04
General surgery	4	5,8%
Orthopedics	2	2,9%
Total	69	100%

To simplify comparison with other studies, hospital wards have been grouped into 4 main categories (Figure 32):

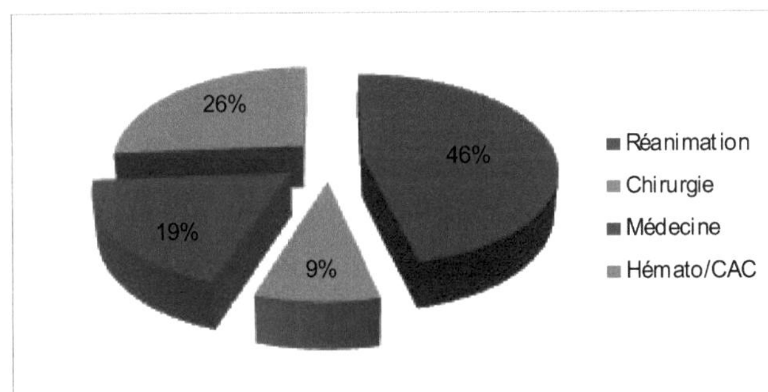

Figure. 32: Distribution of CS cases in the 4 main types of department (Intensive Care, Surgery, Hematology-CAC, Medicine)

- Intensive care (all intensive care units, including medical and surgical intensive care).

- Surgery (all surgeries combined).

- Hematology and CAC.

- Medicine, bringing together all the other departments concerned (Internal Medicine, Nephrology).

12.4 Annual breakdown of CS cases

The distribution of CS cases by year during the study period is shown in (Figure 33).

The average annual number of CS cases is around 23, but there are disparities from one year to the next, with a significant increase in 2017 with 40 cases and a marked decrease in 2018 with only 8 cases diagnosed.

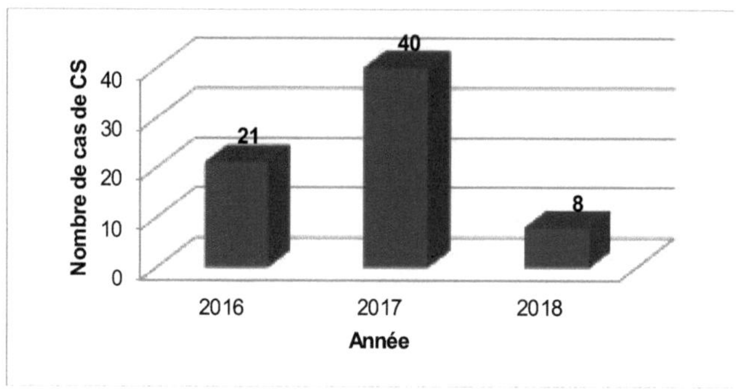

Figure. 33: Annual distribution of CS cases during the study period

12.5   Cumulative incidence or attack rate calculated by year

✓ **Year 2016**

During 2016, 8800 patients were hospitalized in the above-mentioned departments. 21 cases of CS were diagnosed. This gives us an incidence of =2.4 per 1000 admissions.

✓ **Year 2017**

During 2017, 9621 patients were hospitalized in the above-mentioned departments. 40 cases of CS were diagnosed. This gives us an incidence of =4.16 per 1000 admissions.

✓ **Year 2018**

During 2018, 7902 patients were hospitalized in the above-mentioned departments. 8 cases of CS were diagnosed. This gives us an incidence of =1.01 per 1000 admissions.

In total during the study period from January 1, 2016 to December 31, 2018, 26323 patients were hospitalized in the above-mentioned departments. 69 cases of CS were diagnosed. This gives us an incidence of =2.62 per 1000 admissions.

12.6 Incidence of CS by hospital ward

Figure. 34, the distribution of the incidence of CS according to hospitalization department.

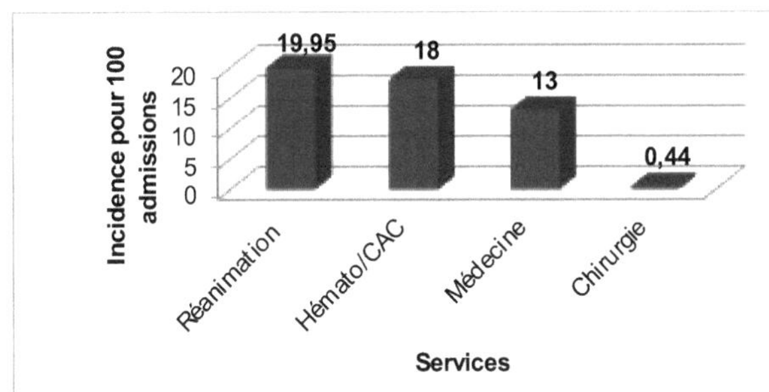

Figure. 34: Incidence of CS by hospital ward

- We note a wide disparity in the distribution of incidences between departments, with a clear predominance in intensive care units (19.95 per 1000 admissions), followed by CAC/Hematology units (18 per 1000 admissions).
- The lowest incidence was recorded in surgical departments (0.44 per 1000 admissions).

12.7 Breakdown of patients by underlying pathology

Table VIII shows the underlying pathologies found in the patients included in our study.

Hematological malignancy was the most frequent underlying pathology in (30%) of patients, followed by chronic renal failure in second place in (17%) of patients, then diabetes in (14%) of patients.

Table VIII: Breakdown of patients by underlying pathology

Underlying pathologies	Number of patients	Frequency
Malignant hemopathy	19	30%
Diabetes	8	14%
Chronic renal failure (CRF)	11	17%
Hepatitis	5	8%

Endocarditis	1	2%
Arterial hypertension (AH)	4	7%
Polyradiculoneuritis	3	5%
Spondylodiscitis	2	3%
Meningo-encephalitis	4	7%
Abcés fessier	1	2%
Solid organ cancer	3	5%

12.8 Reasons for hospitalization

Figure. 35 shows the distribution of patients by reason for hospitalization.

- Hematological malignancies and septic shock are the most frequent reasons for hospitalization.

- The other patterns are detailed in (Figure 35).

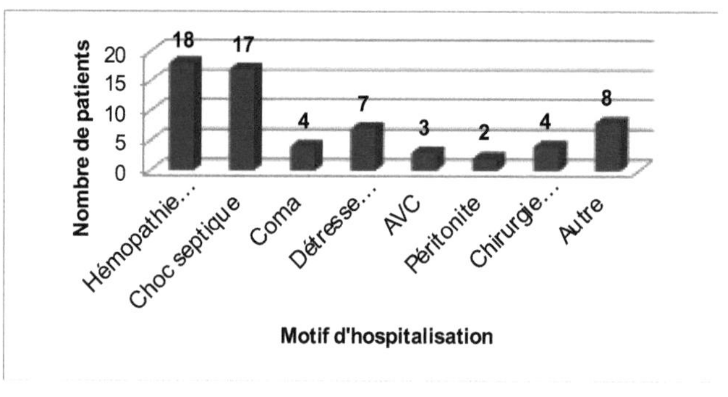

Fig. 35: Distribution of patients by reason for hospitalization

12.9 Risk factors

Various risk factors for CS were investigated using the information collection forms in the clinical records of the patients included in our study.

Table. IX, the various risk factors investigated in our patients.

In our study, the main risk factors found were :

- The existence of prior *Candida spp* colonization at at least 2 peripheral sites was found in all our patients. This colonization can be explained by a stay of ≥ 7 days in (84.12%) of patients, and broad-spectrum antibiotic therapy in (92.06%) of patients. These two risk factors favor the transition from the saprophytic to the pathogenic state, leading to proliferation and colonization.

- The presence of a venous catheter (VC) in (76.19%) of patients.

- Age ≥ 60 years (39.68%).

- Chemotherapy was used in 31.74% of patients.

- A bladder catheter was found in 30.15% of patients.

- Hematological malignancy and neutropenia are two closely related factors found in (28.57%) of patients.

- Other risk factors are detailed in (Table IX).

Table. IX: All risk factors identified in the patients included in our study

Risk factor	Number of patients	Frequency
Age ≥ 60	25	39,68%
Stay ≥7days	53	84,12%
Venous catheter (CV)	48	76,19%
Dialysis	7	11,11%
Neutropenia	18	28,57%
Corticosteroid therapy	13	20,63%
Chemotherapy	20	31,74%
Broad-spectrum antibiotics	58	92,06%
Recent surgery	8	12,69%
Recent digestive surgery	8	12,69%
Immunosuppressive therapy	11	17,46%
Malignant hemopathy	18	28,57%
Colonization ≥ 2 sites	63	100%
Mechanical ventilation	16	25,39%
Bladder probe	19	30,15%

12.10 Colonization index

We report the values of the colonization index calculated in our patients on the (Table. X)

A total of 63 colonization indexes (CI) were calculated.

Based on the threshold value of positivity (CI $\geq$ 0.5), patients were divided into two groups:

- **Group 1**: 14 patients (22.22%) were mildly or moderately colonized: (CI< 0.5).
- **Group 2**: 49 patients (77.78%) were highly colonized (CI$\geq$ 0.5).

Table. X: Calculated colonization index values

Colonization index	Workforce	Percentage
1/5(0,2)	0	0%
2/5(0,4)	14	22,22%
3/5(0,6)	24	38,09%
4/5(0,8)	25	39,68%
5/5(1)	0	0%

12.11 Multivariate analysis of risk factors according to degree of fungal colonization

In Table. XI, we report the results of the multivariate analysis of risk factors according to the degree of fungal colonization.

Table. XI: Multivariate analysis of risk factors according to degree of fungal colonization

	IC< 0.5(14)	IC$\geq$ 0.5(49)	P
Age$\geq$60	10	15	0,005
Stay $\geq$7days	10	43	0,14

Venous catheter (CV)	13	35	0,09
Dialysis	2	5	0,66
Neutropenia	5	13	0,50
Corticosteroid therapy	3	10	0,93
Chemotherapy	9	11	0,003
Broad-spectrum antibiotic therapy	13	45	0,90
Recent surgery	2	6	0,91
Recent digestive surgery	7	1	2
Immunosuppressive therapy	5	6	0,04
Malignant hemopathy	3	15	0,50
Solid organ transplantation	1	4	0,90
Mechanical ventilation	6	10	0,08
Bladder probe	5	14	0,60

12.12 Mycological data

12.12.1 Overall species distribution in deep samples

Table XII shows the distribution of *Candida* species in the various deep samples.

- We obtained 75 *Candida spp* isolates from the cultures of the various deep samples.
- *Non-albicans* species predominate, 45/75 (60%) compared with *Candida albicans* species, 30/75 (40%).
- *Candida parapsilosis* was the *non-albicans* species most frequently isolated (32/45), i.e. (71.11%).

Table. XII: Distribution of *Candida* species in deep samples

	Cm	Pn	Mn	Ar	Ed	%	P
C albicans (n=30)	25	3	2	0	0	40%	0,69
C parapsilosis (n=32)	28	2	1	1	0	42,66%	0,49
C tropicalis (n=8)	5	2	0	0	1	10,66%	0,02
Cglabrata (n=1)	1	0	0	0	0	1,33%	0,99
C krusei (n=4)	3	1	0	0	0	5,33%	0,89

Cm: Candidemia, **Pn:** Peritonitis, **Mn**: Meningitis, **Ar :** Arthritis, **Ed**: Endocarditis, **%:** Percentage, **P:** Chi2.

12.12.2 Peripheral sampling

12.12.2.1 Positive peripheral sampling

In Table XIII, we report the positivity rate of peripheral samples.

Table XIII: Positivity of peripheral samples

	Workforce	Percentage
Peripheral sampling (+)	146	46,35%
Peripheral withdrawals (-)	169	53,65
Total	315	100%

For all 63 patients included in our study, 315 samples from peripheral sites (Buccal, Nasal, Auricular, Urinary and Rectal) were taken, at a rate of 05 samples per patient. Of these samples, 146 were positive for *Candida spp*, representing a positivity rate of (46.35%).

12.12.2.2 Distribution of *Candida* species in positive peripheral samples

Table XIV shows the distribution of *Candida* species in positive peripheral samples.

- In all superficial samples, the proportion of *Candida albicans* did not exceed 50% (39.72%) compared with *non-albicans* species (60.28%).

- *Candida glabrata* was the *non-albicans* species most frequently isolated (43/88), i.e. (48.86%),

Table XIV: Distribution of *Candida* species in positive peripheral samples

	B (n=53)	N (n=17)	A (n=18)	U (n=31)	R (n=27)	%	P
C albicans	21	7	3	10	17	39,72%	0,02
C glabrata	12	6	8	11	6	29,45%	0,32
C	0	0	5	8	3	10,95%	0.
C krusei	2	0	0	1	1	2,74%	0,85

| *C tropicalis* | 18 | 4 | 2 | 1 | 0 | 17,12% | 0. |

B: Buccal, **N**: Nasal, **A:** Auricular, **U**: Urinary, **R**: Rectal, **P**: Chi2

12.12.3   Species distribution by year

Figure. 36, Species distribution by year.

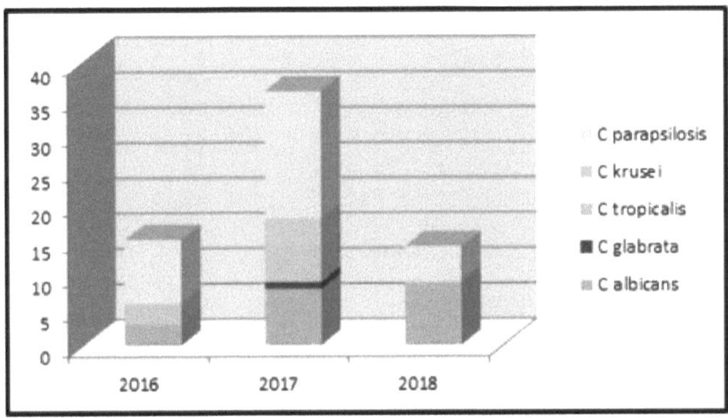

Figure. 36: Species distribution by year

- In 2016 (n=12, 80%) and 2017 (n=28, 60.87%), *non-albicans* species were isolated in the majority compared with *Candida albicans*.
- A decline in the isolation of *non-albicans / Candida albicans* species in 2018 (n= 5, 35.71%,) with the disappearance of *C tropicalis, C krusei* and *Cglabrata* species.
- *C parapsilosis* is the *non-albicans* species most frequently isolated, whatever the year of the study.

12.12.4   Species distribution according to the 4 main service types s

We report on (Table. XV, Figure. 37) the distribution of species according to the 4 main types of service.

Table. XV: Species distribution according to the 4 main service types

	Med **(n=13)**	**Chirg** **(n=10)**	**Hemato/CA** **C** **(n=18)**	**Réa** **(n=34)**	**%**	**P**
C albicans	10	3	4	13	40%	0,01

C *parapsilosis*	3	3	12	14	42,66%	0,07
C tropicalis	0	1	2	5	10,66%	0,54
C krusei	0	1	0	0	1,33%	0,08
C glabrata	0	2	0	2	5,35%	0,11

Med: Medicine, **Chirg**: Surgery, **Hemato/CAC:** Hematology/CAC, **ICU:** Intensive Care Unit, **%**: Percentage, **P=Khi2**.

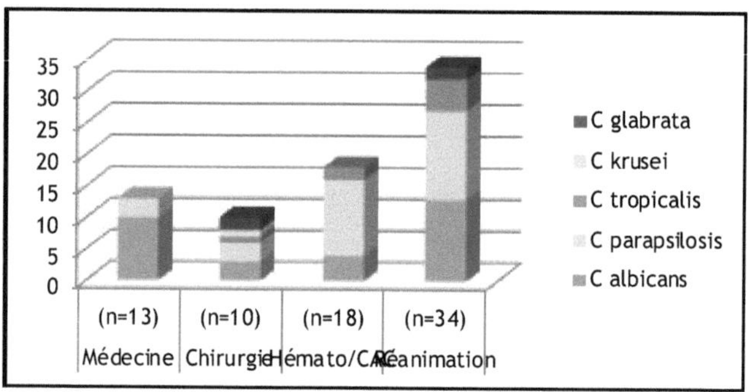

Figure. 37: Species distribution according to the 4 main service types

12.12.5 Underlying pathology

In Figure. 38, the distribution of species in patients with hematological malignancies.

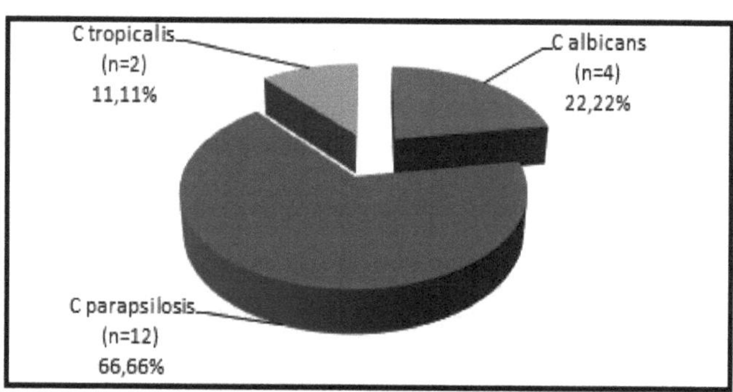

Figure. 38: Species distribution in patients with haematological malignancies

12.12.6   Distribution of *Candida* species according to patient age

Figure. 39, the distribution of *Candida* species according to patient age.

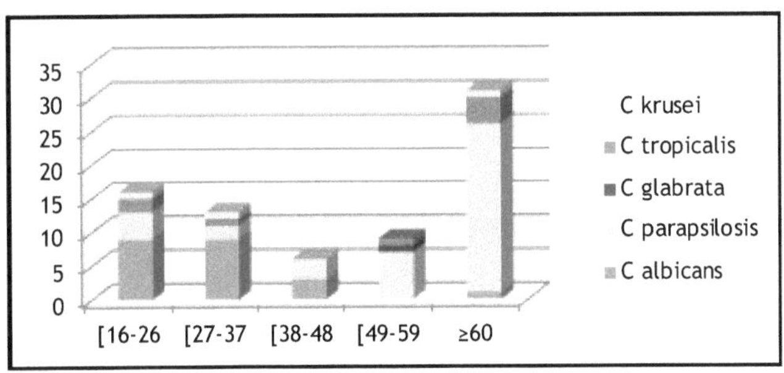

Figure. 39: Distribution of *Candida* species according to patient age

From Figure. 39 we note that :

- Between ages [16-37], *C albicans* species predominates over *non-albicans* species.
- From age 49 onwards, *non-albicans* species predominate *over C albicans* species.
- *C parapsilosis* is the *non-albicans* species most frequently isolated in all age groups.

12.13   Therapeutic management

12.13.1   Antifungal treatment

We report on Table. XVI, the various antifungal agents administered as first-line treatments for systemic candidiasis.

Table. XVI: Different antifungal agents used as first-line treatment for systemic candidiasis

	Caspofungin	Fluconazole	Voriconazole	No
Candidemia	9	3	24	23
Peritonitis	1	3	0	1
Arthritis	0	0	1	0
Meningitis	0	0	3	0
Endocarditi	0	0	1	0
Total	10	6	29	24

Percentage	14,49%	8,7%	42,03%	34,78%

12.13.2 Removal of the venous line

In our study, 48 / 63 patients had a venous line.

Table XVII shows the evolution of patients according to whether or not the venous line was removed.

Table. XVII: Evolution of patients according to whether or not the VV was removed

	VV Ablation	**No VV ablation**
Survival	12(75%)	4(25%)
Deaths	9(28,12%)	23(71,87%)

- Removal of the venous line is associated with the highest survival rate (75%).
- Failure to remove the venous line was associated with the highest mortality rate (71.87%).

12.14 Overall evolution after a positive diagnosis

Figure. 40, the overall evolution after a positive diagnosis:

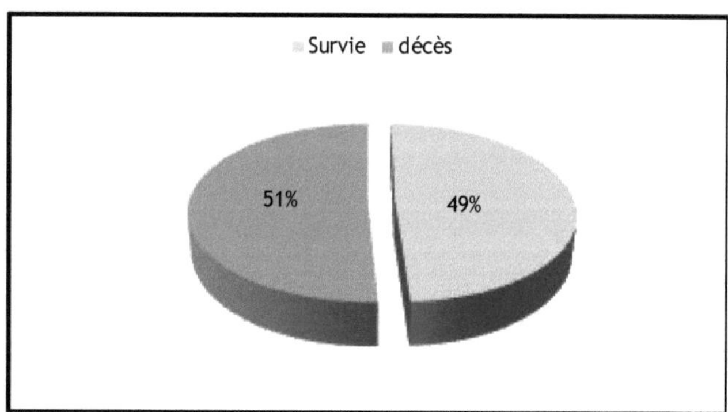

Figure. 40: Overall evolution after positive diagnosis

Progression was favorable for (31/63) patients (49%), and unfavorable for (32/63) patients (51%), leading to death.

12.14.1 Overall patient trends by species

Table XVIII shows the overall evolution of patients according to species.

Table. XVIII: Overall evolution of patients according to species

	C albicans	*C parapsilosis*	*C tropicalis*	*C glabrata*	*C krusei*
Survival	18(43,90%)	16(39,02%)	5(12,19%)	0(0%)	2(4,87%)
Deaths	12(33,33%)	16(44,44%)	3(8,33%)	1(2,77%)	2(5,55%)
P	0,04	0,48	0,63	0,26	0,84

- *C parapsilosis* is associated with the highest mortality rate of 44.44%.
- *C albicans* is associated with the highest survival rate (43.90%).

12.14.2 Overall mortality as a function of treatment

In Figure. 41, the overall mortality of patients according to the treatment received.

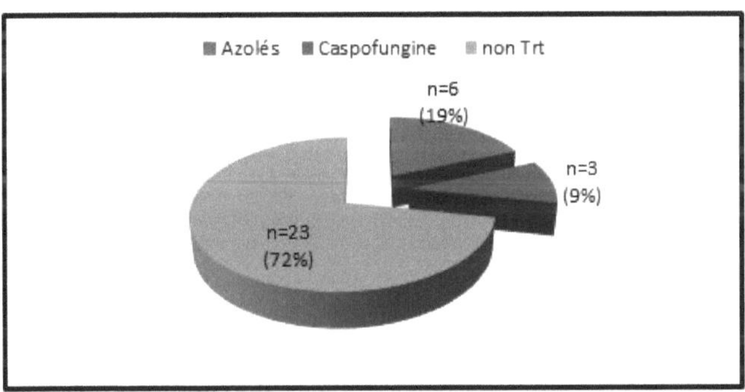

Figure. 41: Overall mortality as a function of treatment received

12.14.3 Overall trend as a function of time to initiation of treatment

Table XIX shows the overall evolution according to the time taken to initiate treatment.

Table. XIX: Overall trend according to time to initiation of treatment

	< 24h	24 - 48h	> 48h	no trt
Surviv ors	19(61,29%)	7(22,58%)	5(16,12%)	0(0%)
Deaths	2(6,25%)	1(3,12%)	6(18,75%)	23(71,87%)
P	3,60	0,02	0,78	3,14

Late initiation of treatment> 48 hours is associated with the highest mortality rate (18.75%), while early initiation< 24 hours yields the highest survival rate (61.29%).

Abstinence from treatment always results in death (71.87%).

12.14.4   Mortality by hospital ward

In Figure. 42, mortality according to hospitalization department:

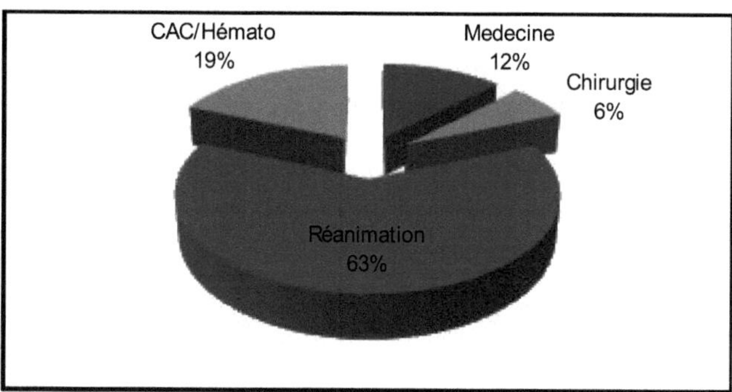

Figure. 42: Mortality by hospital ward

Intensive care units had the highest mortality rate (63%) compared to other units.

12.14.5   Overall trend by patient age

In Figure. 43, Overall evolution as a function of patient age.

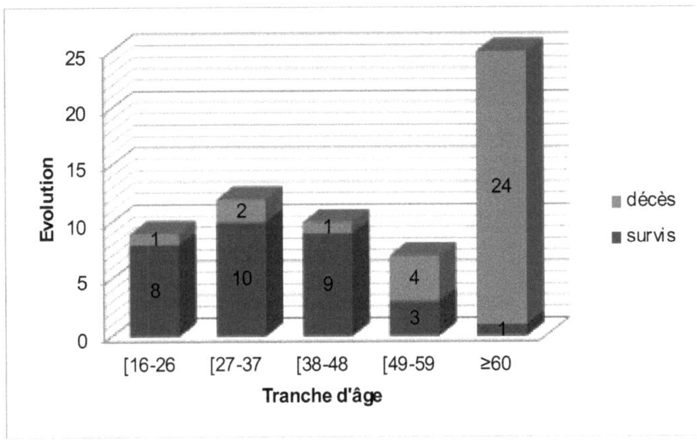

Fig. 43: Overall trends by patient age

12.15   Interest of mannan antigenemia and anti-mannan antibodies assays
in the diagnosis of CS

Patients included in this part of the study are classified into two groups:

➢   **Group 1**

60 patients had proven deep-lying candidiasis (positive blood culture or another *Candida-positive* deep-lying sample)

➢   **Group 2**

26 patients were colonized by *Candida spp* (unproven candidiasis).

Table. XX: Performance of antigenemia alone

Antigenemia	Patients with CSP	Colonized patients
Positive	24	00
Negative	36	26

Sensitivity: 40% of the time

Specificity: 100%.

Table. XXI: Performance of serology alone

Serology	Patients with CSP	Colonized patients
Positive	7	4
Negative	53	22

Sensitivity: 11.67

Specificity: 84.62

Table. XXII: Performance of antigenemia and associated serology

Antigenemia δ Serology	Patients with CSP	Colonized patients
Ag and/or Ac positive	29	4
Negative Ag and Ac	30	22

Sensitivity: 49.15

Specificity: 84.62

13 DISCUSSION

The main aim of this prospective bicentric study is to assess the epidemiology of systemic candidiasis and its evolution over time at BATNA University Hospital and CAC.

In fact, most studies of systemic candidiasis, whether national or international, are multicentric and vary from one center to another, from one region to another and from one country to another, hence the interest in these studies for gaining insight into local epidemiology, despite the disadvantage that the number of cases reported is small, making it necessary to carry out long-term studies.

One of the strong points of our study is that the mycological examination was carried out in our Parasitology-Mycology laboratory, which enabled us to systematically include all patients with deep samples positive for *Candida spp* and their immediate examination in order to determine the species involved in a codified manner. This study, which took place over a three-year period from January 1, 2016 to December 31, 2018, resulted in the isolation of 69 proven cases of systemic candidiasis in 63 patients, involving 75 isolates.

13.1 Demographics

13.1.1 Average age

In our study, the mean age was 48.31 years. According to several studies, the ages most at risk of systemic candidiasis are often between 50 and 65 [229,230].

David L Horn et al found a mean age of 53.5 years [229]. Matteo Bassetti et al (2013) found a mean age of 66.2 years [230]. In contrast, Khelfaoui et al (2016) found a mean age of 29.24 years [231].

13.1.2 Sex ratio

In terms of gender distribution, we noted a predominance of males (65%), with a sex ratio M/F =1.86, which is in line with all the data published to date.

In an American study (2004 -2008) of 2019 patients, 1084 were men, i.e. (53.5%) of all patients [229]. This clear male predominance is also found in other studies: Gupta et al 2015 (57.76%) [232], Bassetti et al 2013 (57%) [230].

On a national scale, Arrache et al (2015) in a study of fungemias diagnosed in the Parasitology-Mycology laboratory at CHU Mustapha in Algiers between (2004-2014), also found a predominance of the male sex (64.61%) with a sex ratio M/F= 1.8 [233]. Khelfaoui et al in a study of invasive candidiasis in the intensive care unit at Constantine University Hospital (2015-2016), found a sex ratio M/F=1.01 [231].

The most likely explanation is that the male population is more represented among patients with major risk factors for systemic candidiasis.

13.2   Risk services

In our study, intensive care units were the units most at risk of CS, with 32/69 cases of CS diagnosed, i.e. (46%). This rate is higher than that reported by Tessier at Bordeaux University Hospital (35%) [234], that reported by Sasso et al (2017) at Nîmes University Hospital (23.3%) [235] and that reported by Tadec et al (2017) at Nantes University Hospital (27.7%) [236].

In second place come the haematology/CAC departments with18/69 cases, i.e. (26%) of all CS cases diagnosed, our result is far from that reported by Tessier (2017) at Bordeaux University Hospital (13%) [234] and that reported by Tadec et al (2016) at Nantes University Hospital (18.8%) [236].

Intensive care and haematology/CAC wards were the most affected by CS; given that they had housed patients with the most risk factors as found (CV, neutropenia, haematological malignancy, chemotherapy, ventilation, broad-spectrum antibiotic therapy, stay$\geq$7 days).

In medical wards, we reported 13/69 cases, i.e. (19%), which is far from the results reported by Tessier (2017) at Bordeaux University Hospital (39%) [234].

The lowest proportion of CS was reported in surgical departments 06 /69 cases i.e. (9%), relatively close to that found by Tessier (2017) at Bordeaux University Hospital (13%) [234]. This low rate is related to the lower number of samples received from surgical departments.

13.3 Incidence

During the study period, 26323 patients were hospitalized in the above-mentioned departments, and 69 cases of CS were diagnosed. This gives an incidence rate of 2.62

per 1000 admissions, which is close to that found in several studies: Nolla-Salas et al (1997) with a rate of 2/1000 admissions [237], Charles et al (2003) with a rate of 2.1/1000 admissions [238] and Colombot al (2006) with a rate of 2.49/1000 admissions [239] (see Table (XXIII).

This incidence is considered high and can be explained by the multiplication of CS risk factors in our hospital.

Table XXIII: Incidence of systemic candidiasis in hospitalized patients

Authors	Observed period	Patient type	Rate/1000 admissions
Nolla-Salas et al. Intensive Care Med. 1997	1995	Resuscitation	2
Charles et al. Intensive Care Med 2003	1990-2000	Resuscitation	2,1
Colombo et al. J Clin Microbiol 2006	2003-2004	The whole hospital	2,49
Our series	2016-2018	The whole hospital	2,62

13.4 Proportion

13.4.1 Candidemia

In our study we received 59 positive blood cultures, corresponding to 59 cases of candidemia, so the proportion of isolated candidemias out of all cases of CS diagnosed was (85.5%). Horn et al (2007) found (77.9%) [240], Lamagni et al (2001) (98%) [2], and Arrache et al (2015) found (92.3%) [233].

Lower proportions than ours were found by Bitar et al (2013), in a study of invasive mycoses in mainland France, the proportion of isolated candidemias was (43.3%) [241].

Leroy et al (2009) (32.1%) [242], and Khelfaoui et al (2016) only (6.04%) [231].

This high proportion can be explained by the frequent use of CVs, a risk factor found in (76.19%) of our patients, especially as the species most frequently isolated from blood cultures was *C parapsilosis*, a species closely linked to the use of CVs.

Table XXIV: Proportion of candidemias among hospitalized patients

Authors	Observed period	Patient type	Proportion
Horn et al. Inf. Dis 2007	2006	The whole hospital	77,9%
Lamagni et al.			98%
Arrache et al. Journal of Medical Mycology 2015	2004-2014	The whole hospital	92,3%
Bitar et al. BHE 2013	2001-2010	All hospitals	43,3%
Leroy et al. Crit Care Med. 2009	2005-2006	All hospitals	32,1%
Khelfoui et al. Thesis2016	2015-2016	Resuscitation	6,04%
Our series	2016-2018	The whole hospital	85,5%

13.4.2 Peritonitis

In our study we received 05 positive peritoneal fluids, corresponding to (7.25%) of all CS diagnosed. This rate is close to that reported by Dupont et al (2003) (10%) [115].

Proportions higher than ours have been reported by: Calandra et al (1989) (42%) [243], Montravers et al (1996) (22%) [244] and Sandven et al (2006) (18%) [245].

Delestre et al (2013) reported only (2%) cases of *Candida spp* peritonitis in the surgical intensive care unit at ROUEN University Hospital [246] (see Table XXV).

The low rate of *Candida spp* peritonitis isolated in our study can be explained by the fact that only (12.69%) of our patients underwent digestive surgery, which is a major risk factor for *Candida spp* peritonitis.

Table XXV: Proportion of peritonitis in hospitalized patients

Authors	Observed period	Patient type	Proportion
Dupont et al. Crit Care Med 2003	1994-1999	Surgical resuscitation	10%
Montravers et al. Clin Infect Dis 1996	1987-1992	Surgery	22%
Sandven et al. J Clin Microbiol. 2006	1991-2003	Surgery	18%
Delestre et al. 2013 thesis	2006-2011	Surgical resuscitation	2%
Our series	2016-2018	The whole hospital	7,25%

13.5 Risk factors

To identify the various risk factors, we relied on those already well identified in the literature. In our series, most patients had multiple risk factors and heavy comorbidities.

CS risk factors can be divided into two groups:

Factors associated with healthcare, including catheter use, parenteral nutrition, surgical procedures and antimicrobial drug use.

Host-related factors include immunosuppressive diseases, neutropenia, age and deterioration of clinical status due to underlying diseases [242, 247, 248,249]

In our study, all the patients included (63 patients) had at least 02 colonized sites, with colonization mainly involving oral (53/146) (36.3%), urinary (31/146) (21.23%) and rectal (27/146) (18.49%) sites. *Candida* colonization is a risk factor whose importance has been recognized in recent years. According to various studies, this risk factor for the development of CS is more related to the presence or absence of colonization than to the number of colonized areas [90,102]. In any case, the absence of *Candida* colonization is a strong indicator in favor of excluding the diagnosis of CS [90,102].

In our study, a prolonged stay≥ 7 days, implies an increased risk of developing CS (found in 53/63 patients or 84.12%), which is in line with a recent publication by Murray et al, who highlighted that the expansion of fungal infection and sepsis was related to the length of hospital stay [250].

Vincent et al (1995) in the EPIC study showed that patients with 21 days or more of hospitalization in the ICU had a 33-fold increase in the risk of acquiring a nosocomial infection, compared with those staying 24 to 48 hours in the same department [92]. Zaoutis et al (2005) showed that systemic candidiasis prolonged the length of stay by an average of 10 days [251].

Exposure to broad-spectrum antibiotics was a risk factor for CS in 58/63 patients (92.06%). Antibiotic treatment was systematic, as septic shock was the most common reason for hospitalization in (33.33%) of our patients.

The risk of fungal complications increases with prolonged, broad-spectrum antibiotic treatment. According to the study by Wey et al (1989), the number of different antibiotics was the most important prognostic risk factor for the expansion of candidiasis, (94%) of patients who developed candidiasis had already been exposed to antibiotics, which is close to our proportion [107].

The breadth of the antimicrobial spectrum and duration of exposure are also correlated with the risk of fungal complication [94]. In our study, over 60% of patients received more than 2 broad-spectrum antibiotics.

Fraser et al (1992), reported that (94%) of patients with candidemia had been previously exposed to antibiotics and (62%) had received more than four different molecules [108].

Antibiotics destroy the commensal microbial flora, releasing muramic acid from the bacterial wall, which leads to yeast filamentation and opportunistic *Candida* proliferation.

In our study, 48/63 patients (76.19%) had a venous catheter, as the majority were hospitalized in the intensive care and hematology/CAC departments. The intravascular catheter used for parenteral nutrition supports the evolution of several *Candida* species [252,253]. When the catheter is inserted, adventitial trauma is created at the entry point, leading to thrombosis. The yeast multiplies in the vicinity of the catheter entry point, then infiltrates the vein and colonizes the pre-existing thrombus. In this way, the thrombus can cause the yeast to spread into the bloodstream, leading to fungal embolisms. Studies have shown that in catheter-associated bloodstream infections, *Candida spp* have a shorter growth time than those from other sources [254].

In our study, neutropenia was found in 18/63 patients (28.57%). Hematological malignancy was found in 18/63 patients (28.57%). Chemotherapy was found in 20/63 patients (31.74%). These three risk factors are very closely linked. Hematological malignancies generate a deficiency of neutrophils (PNN), which are essential to the body's defense against yeast dissemination. Neutropenia can also occur during treatment of leukemia with cytostatic drugs or immunosuppressants used to prevent rejection of bone marrow or kidney transplants.

Our study did not identify recent surgery as a predominant risk factor; it was only found in 08 patients (12.69%). This compares with the study by Tortorano et al (2006), who found recent surgery in (50%) of cases [255].

Several studies have shown the relationship between candidemia and recent surgery [256,257], especially abdominal surgery. There are several explanations for this observation, but manipulation of the intestine, and the effect of resection on intestinal microbiology, microbiota abundance and epithelial function could contribute to the possibility of candidemia. Studies have shown that patients with high anastomotic leakage, as well as those with recurrent gastrointestinal perforation, acute necrotizing pancreatitis, present a higher risk of candidemia [111].

Multivariate analysis of risk factors according to the degree of fungal colonization revealed that age ≥60 years **(P=0.005)**, chemotherapy **(P=0.003)** and immunosuppressive treatment **(P=0.04)** were the risk factors most significantly associated with the risk of developing systemic candidiasis in highly colonized patients (CI ≥0.5).

13.6 Mycological data

C. albicans was traditionally the most isolated species. However, a trend towards *non-albicans* species has been observed worldwide over the past 15 years. In our study, we obtained 75 isolates from different deep cultures. Species identification revealed a predominance of *non-albicans* species (45/75 isolates or 60%) compared with *Candida albicans* species (30/75 isolates or 40%), which is in line with several studies [233,258, 262,263]. In other studies, however, *Candida albicans* was the most frequently isolated species, compared with *non-albicans* [231, 245,259].

As in all studies published to date other than *Candida albicans, C parapsilosis, C tropicalis, C krusei* and *C glabrata* were isolated.

In our study, *C parapsilosis* was the most frequently isolated *non-albicans* species, 32/75 isolates or 42.66%, which is not usually found in the literature where *C. glabrata* is the most commonly isolated [260,261].

On the other hand, several studies found a predominance of this species in all isolates. Arrache et al 2016 isolated *C parapsilosis* with a frequency of (36.6%) [233], Ng et al (2001) (51%) [262], Khalfaoui (2016) (22.22%) [231], and Medrano et al (2006) (36%) [263] and Montagna (2013) (43.84%) [258].

Table XXVI: Distribution of *Candida* species

	P Sandven 2006 [245]	MT Montagna 2013 [258]	N Yapar 2011 [259]	N Khelfaoui 2015-2016 [231]	D Arrache 2015 [233]	DJ Medrano 2006 [263]	KP Ng 2001 [262]	Our series

C albicans	70%	40,2%	45,8%	55,55%	31,6%	28%	11,8%	40%
C glabrata	13%	7,98%	4,8%	/	/	4%	1%	1,33%
C parpsilosis	6%	43,84%	14,5%	22,22%	36,6%	36%	51%	42,66%
C tropicalis	7%	7,98%	24,1%	22,22%	23,3%	16%	25,5%	10,66%
C krusei	/	/		/	3,3%	/	/	5,35%

C. parapsilosis is more frequently associated with the presence of a central venous line and the use of parenteral nutrition than any other fungal species [264].

He emphasized that *C parapsilosis* is a frequent skin colonizer and is often associated with catheter-related infections. Parenteral nutrition and endocarditis in cardiac surgery patients [265,266].

(46%) of the patients included in our study were hospitalized in intensive care and (26%) in hematology/CAC, (76.19%) of whom had a venous catheter, which could explain the greater frequency of this species.

In patients with solid tumors and candidemia at the University of Texas M. D. Anderson Cancer Center between 1998 and 2002, the rates of candidemia caused by *C. albicans* and *C. parapsilosis* were 40% and 35% respectively [267].

In contrast, an earlier study indicated that *C. parapsilosis* accounted for only 7% of *Candida* infections in oncology patients [268].

The use of broad-spectrum antibiotics favours the emergence *of C parapsilosis* [201]. 92.06% of our patients had received broad-spectrum antibiotics (Vancomycin, Emipinem, Tienam, Ertoperene, Ciprolon, Amikacin).

In vitro, *C. parapsilosis* has a significantly lower level of sensitivity to echinocandins (Caspofungin, Anidulafungin, Micafungin) than other *Candida* species. The introduction of Caspofungin coincided with the emergence of *C. parapsilosis* candidemia, with a tendency to be linked to its level of consumption in intensive care units [201].

C tropicalis ranked third among *Candida* isolates, with 8/75 isolates (10.66%), in line with studies [255,269]. This low rate can be explained by the fact that our population is young≥ 16 years and this species is frequently isolated from children and newborns [214, 247]. Arrache et al (2015) isolated *C tropicalis* in 23.3% of isolates [233].

We isolated *Candida krusei* in 4/75 isolates (5.33%); in 4 patients with food poisoning from a dairy product admitted to intensive care. Data found in some studies [233, 270,271].

By calculating the Chi2 (see Table XII)

- *C tropicalis* is the species most significantly isolated from blood cultures **P=0.02**.
- There is no significant difference in isolation from other species.

Of all positive surface samples, *Candida albicans* presented 58/146 or (39.72%) compared to *non-albicans* species with 88/146 or (60.28%).

Candida glabrata was the *non-albicans* species most frequently isolated (43/88), i.e. (48.86%).

By calculating the Chi2 (see Table XIV) :

- *C albicans* is the species most significantly isolated from buccal swabs **P=0.02**.
- *C parapsilosis* is the species most significantly isolated in urine samples **P=0.0003.**
- *C tropicalis* is the species most significantly isolated from buccal samples **P=0.0002**.
- For other species, there is no significant difference in isolation.

Distribution of *Candida* species according to patient age from Fig. 39 we note that:

- Between ages [16-37], *C albicans* species predominates over *non-albicans* species.
- From age 49, *non-albicans* species predominate *over C albicans* species.
- *C parapsilosis* is the *non-albicans* species most frequently isolated in all age groups.

The majority of isolates were obtained from intensive care units (34/75) (45.33%), and haematology/CAC (18/75) (24%).

By calculating the Chi2 (see Table XV), *C albicans* is the species most significantly isolated in intensive care units **P=0.01**.

13.7 Underlying pathologies

Hematological malignancy was the most common underlying pathology (18/63 patients, or 30%). All patients were hospitalized in hematology/CAC wards, with a clear predominance of *non-albicans* species (14/18) (77.78%) compared with *Candida albicans* species (4/18) (22.22%). (Figure42)

Candida parapsilosis was the *non-albicans* species most frequently isolated (12/14), i.e. (85.71%).

According to his results, the underlying pathology is closely linked to species distribution. In our study, patients with hematological malignancies were more likely to develop candidemia to *non-albicans* species (*C parapsilosis*) than to *Candida albicans* species.

13.8 Therapeutic management

13.8.1 Antifungal treatment

We report on Table. XVI, the various antifungal agents administered as first-line treatments for systemic candidiasis.

- Regarding antifungal treatment, 35 cases of CS or 50.72% were treated with azoles, mainly **Voriconazole** (29 cases or 42.03%) and 6 cases or 8.7% were treated with Fluconazole.
- Caspofungin was used to treat 10 cases of CS (14.49%).
- 24 CS cases (34.78%) were not treated.

- **Voriconazole** was therefore the molecule most frequently used to treat CS cases in our study.

13.8.2 Removal of the venous line

In our study, 48/63 patients had a venous line (Table XVII).

Removal of the venous catheter (VV) is a good prognostic factor. A 75% survival rate is associated with removal of the venous catheter.

Failure to remove the venous line is associated with high mortality (71.87%).

Therefore, non-removal of the venous line is a risk factor for mortality, and the Chi2 calculation is highly significant, **P=0.002**.

13.9 Overall trends and mortality

The outcome was favorable for (31/63) patients, i.e. (49%), and unfavorable for (32/63) patients, i.e. (51%), culminating in death, giving a high mortality rate underscoring the seriousness of these infections (Figure40).

Our mortality rate is high compared with that found by Horn (2009) (35.2%) [229], Xavier Tessier (2017) and Khalfaoui et al (2016) (33.3%) [231,234].

The high mortality rate in our study is explained by :

- Delayed diagnosis, sometimes even in the post-mortem phase or in severe sepsis.
- Delayed initiation of antifungal treatment >48 hours.
- The choice of antifungal treatment is based on the molecule available in the hospital, rather than on the sensitivity of the species in question.
- Neglect of antifungal treatment despite a positive diagnosis.
- Non-compliance with treatment duration (14 days after the last positive blood culture).

In our study, we were able to demonstrate certain factors influencing the mortality rate:

- The *Candida* species involved: *C parapsilosis* is associated with a poorer prognosis, with over 44% of patients presenting an unfavorable evolution.
  In contrast, patients with *C albicans* have the highest survival rate (43.90%) (Table

XVIII).

By calculating the Chi2, *C albicans* is the species most significantly associated with a good prognosis **P=0.04**.

- Wards housing high-risk CS patients had very high mortality rates, as in our study, intensive care units had the highest mortality rates compared with other wards, accounting for over half of all deaths (63%) (Figure42).

- Advanced age ≥60 years is correlated with poor prognosis and high mortality 24/32 deaths or 75% (Figure43).

- Failure to institute treatment was responsible for a high mortality rate of 23/32 deaths (72%) (Figure41).

  The choice of treatment determines the outcome, with more deaths observed with the use of azoles (06/32 deaths or 19%) than with the use of echinocandins (Caspofungin) (03/32 deaths or 9%)(Figure41).

  Initial use of azoles is associated with a higher mortality rate than Echinocandins. According to some studies, echinocandins are more effective than azoles in the treatment of invasive candidiasis [272, 273,274], which is in line with our results.

- The time taken to initiate antifungal treatment has a decisive influence on the outcome. It is interesting to note that the time taken to initiate treatment has a major influence on patient outcome. Thus, late initiation of treatment> 48 hours is associated with the highest mortality rate (18.75%), while early initiation< 24 hours yields the highest survival rate (61.29%). Abstinence from treatment always results in death (72%) (Table XIX).

  When the Chi2 is calculated, administration of antifungal treatment within 24-48 hours is most significantly associated with a good prognosis **(P=0.02).**

- Failure to remove the venous line is associated with high mortality (**P=0.002**). (Table XVII).

  The same observation was made by (Beraud 2009) with a calculated Chi2 =0.038 [275] Rex et al have shown that catheter removal shortens the duration of candidemia [276]. Patients with catheter-related infections have a higher inoculum, which explains the faster time to development and the fact that observational studies have shown lower mortality when the catheter is removed [277,278].

13.10   The value of Mn antigen and antibody assays

- The proportion of patients with positive Mn antigenemia and proven CS is (40%).
  The same proportion was observed by Sendid [279].

  The proportion of patients with negative Mn antigenemia and no proven CS
  (colonized) is (100%).

  The Mn antigen assay alone can therefore be used to differentiate between infected
  and colonized patients (Table XX).

- The proportion of patients with positive serology and proven CS is (11.67%).

  The proportion of patients with negative serology and no proven CS (colonized) is
  (84.62%).

  So serology alone cannot differentiate between infected and colonized patients
  (low sensitivity) (Tableua XXI).

- The combination of the two tests resulted in an increase in sensitivity (49.15%)
  with a specificity of (84.62%); our result is very far from the sensitivities observed
  in various studies. Sendid et al (84%) [279].

  So the combination of the two tests enables us to differentiate between infected
  and colonized patients (Table XXII).

13.11 Study limits

Our study had a number of limitations:

- A small sample size necessitates a multi-year study.
- Requesting mycological examinations of deep samples, including blood cultures,
  is not a reflex for clinicians, which minimized the size of our study sample. Each
  time, we had to go to the wards and make clinicians aware of the value of
  mycological diagnosis.
- The limitation of our sample was also due to the fact that patients were
  systematically treated with antifungal agents, even in the absence of clinical signs
  (as a prophylactic measure).
- We were confronted with the non-availability of diagnostic tools, whether
  biological or serological, and self-financing was the only way to carry out this
  study.
- The lack of collaboration on the part of some clinicians, especially with regard to

treatment initiation and adherence to treatment duration, and even the release of patients without antifungal coverage, had an impact on our results and evolution.

CONCLUSION/ RECOMMENDATIONS

Our prospective epidemiological study was carried out over a three-year period at BATNA's CHU and CAC. We were able to identify the different *Candida* species involved, the risk factors predisposing to contracting this infection and the factors influencing prognosis.

Systemic candidiasis remains a severe condition, and one that is constantly on the increase, due to the growing number of people at risk. A high incidence was recorded in our study (2.62 per 1000 admissions), in line with international data, which underlines the importance of these conditions. Their prognosis remains very poor, due on the one hand to the severity of the condition itself, which is responsible for a high mortality rate (51%) (a very high rate compared with national or even international data), and on the other hand to the severity of the underlying pathologies. In our study, haematological malignancy was the underlying pathology most predisposing to the risk of systemic candidiasis, which led us to give greater importance to looking for these infections in patients hospitalized in oncology/haematology with leukemia, especially in the presence of clinical signs that allow a pre-emptive diagnosis.

Several risk factors predispose to CS: endogenous colonization favored by broad-spectrum antibiotic therapy, the degree of colonization by *Candida* yeasts, neutropenia, the use of multiple invasive procedures (CV), advanced age, chemotherapy, prolonged stay... etc. Therefore, knowledge of the risk factors and the profile of patients most at risk of CS, especially in intensive care and haematology/CAC departments, is one of the means of guiding us towards a presumptive diagnosis, and enabling us to initiate pre-emptive treatment in order to reduce the mortality rate.

In the case of systemic (biologically proven) candidiasis, curative treatment adapted to the patient's immune status and the sensitivity of isolated strains to antifungal agents must be instituted as quickly as possible (< 24 hours), while respecting the recommended duration and dose, to avoid therapeutic failure and the emergence of resistance. Specific treatment is now consensual, based on the first-line use of an Echinocandin.

We strongly recommend removing the source of the :

- Systematic removal of venous catheters (VCs).
- Avoid random and abusive use of broad-spectrum antibiotics for fever.
- We recommend starting with a monotherapy adapted to the antibiogram.
- Have the reflex to suspect systemic candidiasis when fever persists beyond 3 days despite appropriate antibiotic therapy.

Finally, to prevent deep-rooted *Candida* infections, we strongly recommend :

- Strict observance of basic hygiene by disinfecting the hands of nursing, medical and paramedical staff using a hydro-alcoholic solution.
- The use of Fluconazole prophylaxis (400mg / day) to reduce the incidence of superficial and systemic *Candida* yeast infections: In neutropenic patients after bone marrow or solid organ transplantation.
  In HIV-infected patients, helps prevent oropharyngeal and esophageal candidiasis In moderately and highly colonized (CI $\geq$ 0.5) intensive care patients with gastrointestinal surgery or acute pancreatitis.

BIBLIOGRAPHY

[1]   Kullberg BJ, Arendrup MC. Invasive candidiasis. N Engl J Med. 2015 Oct 8,373(15): 1445-56.

[2]   Lamagni TL, Evans BG, Shigematsu M, et al. Emerging trends in the epidemiology of invasive mycoses in England and Wales (1990 -9). Epidemiol Infect 2001: 126: 397-414.

[3]   Wisplinghoff H, Bischoff T, Tallent SM, et al. Nosocomial bloodstream infections in US hospitals: Analysis of 24179 cases from a prospective nation-wide surveillance study. Clin Infect Dis 2004: 39: 309-3172.

[4]   Marchetti O, Bille J, Fluckiger U, and al. Epidemiology of candidemia in Swiss tertiary care hospitals: Secular trends, 1991-2000. Clin Infect Dis 2004:38: 311-3203.

[5]   Lepape A. Candidoses graves en réanimation. In: BLANLOEIL Y, eds. Conférences d'actualisation 1999, 41ème Congrès national d'anesthésie et de réanimation. Paris, Elsevier, 1999: 495-503.

[6]   Ascioglu S, Rex JH, de Pauw B, Bennett JE, Bille J, Crokaert F, et al. Defining opportunistic invasive fungal infections in immunocompromised patients with cancer and hematopoietic stem cell transplants: an international consensus. Clin Infect Dis. 2002 Jan 1:34(1): 7-14.

[7]   Eggimann P, Garbino J, Pittet D. Epidemiology of Candida species infections in critically ill non-immunosuppressed patients. Lancet Infect Dis 2003; 11: 685-702.

[8]   Oberoi JK. Invasive candidiasis. JIMSA January - March 2010 Vol. 23 No. 1.

[9]   Yapar N. Epidemiology and risk factors for invasive candidiasis. Ther Clin Risk Manag. 2014; 10:95-105.

[10]   Sendid B, Poirot JL, Tabouret M, Bonnin A, Caillot D, Camus D, et al. Combined detection of mannanemia and antimannan antibodies as a strategy for the diagnosis of systemic infection caused by pathogenic Candida species. J Med Microbiol. 2002; 51(5): 433-42

[11]   Almirante B, Rodriguez D, Park BJ, Cuenca-Estrella M, Planes AM, Almela M, et al. Epidemiology and predictors of mortality in cases of Candida bloodstream infection: results from population-based surveillance, Barcelona Spain, from 2002 to 2003. J Clin Microbiol, 43 (2005), pp. 1829-1835.

[12] Chabasse D. Molds of medical interest. Cahier de formation biologie médicale March 2002.

[13] Lusven M, Poedras LE. MEDICAL MYCOLOGY: Classification of organisms. Parasitology, medical mycology, Guiguen 14/09/2010.

[14] Buffo J, Herman MA and Soll DR. A characterization of pH-regulated dimorphism in Candida albicans. Mycopathologia. 1984. 85 :21-30.

[15] http: //www. botany. hawaii. edu/faculty/wong/BOT135/DESCRIPT. htm

[16] https: //cienciaybiologia. com/subdivision-zygomycotina

[17] http: //www. microbiologiemedicale. fr

[18] http://sites.google. com/site/plantevolutionarydiversity/basidiomycota-agaricomycotina

[19] www.microbiologiemedicale.fr/mycologie/classificationdeschampignonsmicr scopiques.htm

[20] Bialkova A and Subik J. Biology of the pathogenic yeast Candida glabrata. Folia Microbiol. 2006. 51: 3&20.

[21] http: //www. microbiologyinpictures. com/bacteria-photos/Candida-albicans-photos/Candida. html

[22] http: //campus. cerimes. fr/parasitologie/enseignement/candidos/site/html/6. html

[23] Sudbery P, Gow N and Berman J. The distinct morphogenic states of Candida albicans. Trends Microbiol 2004. 12: 317-324.

[24] Barelle CJ, Richard ML, Gaillardin C, Gow NA and Brown AJ. Candida albicans VAC8 is required for vacuolar inheritance and normal hyphal branching. Eukaryot Cell. 2006 Feb; 5(2): 359-67.

[25] http: //archive. bio. ed. ac. uk/jdeacon/FungalBiology/chap16_i. htm

[26]   Gow NA. Candida albicans switches mates. Mol Cell 2002. 10: 217-218.

[27] Cole GT, Seshan KR, Phaneuf M and Lynn KT. Chlamydospore-like cells of Candida albicans in the gastrointestinal tract of infected immunocompromised mice. Can J Microbiol 1991. 37: 637-646.

[28] http: //nursingcrib. com/microbiology/candida-albicans/

[29]   Kibbler CC, Seaton S, Barnes RA and al. Management and outcome of bloodstream infections due to Candida species in England and Wales. J Hosp Infect. 2003; 54(1): 18-24.

[30]   Anane A, Kallel K, Kaouech E, BelHaj S, Chaker E. Candida dubliniensis: a new emerging species. Annales de biologie clinique volume 65 number 1 January-February 2007.

[31]   Forche A, Schönian G, Gräser Y, Vilgalys R, Mitchell TG. 1999. Genetic structure of typical and atypical populations of Candida albicans from Africa. Fungal Genet. Biol. 28: 107-125.

[32]   Tietz HJ, Küssner A, Thanos M, De Andrade MP, Presber W, Schönian G. 1995. Phenotypic and genotypic characterization of unusual vaginal isolates of Candida albicans from Africa. J. Clin. Microbiol. 33: 2462-2465.

[33]   Alonso-Vargas R, Elorduy L, Eraso E, Cano FJ, Guarro J, Ponton J, Quindos G. 2008. Isolation of Candida africana, probable atypical strains of Candida albicans, from a patient with vaginitis. Med. Mycol. 46: 167-170.

[34]   Jacobsen MD, Boekhout T, Odds FC. 2008. Multilocus sequence typing confirms synonymy but highlights differences between Candida albicans and Candida stellatoidea. FEMS Yeast Res. 8: 764-770.

[35]   Romeo O, De Leo F, Criseo G. 2011. Adherence ability of Candida africana: a comparative study with Candida albicans and Candida dubliniensis. Mycoses 54: e57-e61.

[36]   Campbell CK, Davey KG, Holmes AD, Szekely A, Warnock DW. 1999. Comparison of the API Candida system with the AUXACOLOR2 system for identification of common yeast pathogens. J. Clin. Microbiol. 37: 821-823.

[37]   Chu WS, Magee BB and Magee PT. Construction of an SfiI macrorestriction map of the Candida albicans genome. J Bacteriol 1993. 175: 6637-6651.

[38]   Poulain D, Feuilhade DE, Chauvin M. Candidoses et levuroses diverse Encycl. Med. Chir (Elsevier, Paris), Maladies infectieuses, 8-602-A-10, 1995, 12 p.

[39]   Latge JP. The cell wall: a carbohydrate armour for the fungal cell. Mol Microbiol 2007; 66: 279-90.

[40]   Biswas S, Van Dijck P, Datta A. Environmental sensing and signal transduction pathways regulating morphopathogenic determinants of Candida albicans. Microbiol Mol Biol Rev 2007; 71: 348-76.

[41]   Smits GJ, Kapteyn JC, Van den Ende H, Klis FM. Cell wall dynamics in yeast. Curr Opin Microbiol 1999; 2: 348-52.

[42]   Calderone RA and Braun PC. Adherence and receptor relationships of Candida albicans. Microbiol Rev 1991. 55: 1-20.

[43]   Nakagawa Y, Ohno N and Murai T. Suppression by Candida albicans beta-glucan of cytokine release from activated human monocytes and from T cells in the presence of monocytes. J Infect Dis 2003. 187: 710-713.

[44]   Shepherd MG. Cell envelope of Candida albicans. Crit Rev Microbiol 1987. 15: 7-25

[45]   Chaffin WL, Lopez-Ribot JL, Casanova M, Gozalbo D and Martinez JP. Cell wall and secreted proteins of Candida albicans: identification, function, and expression. Microbiol Mol Biol Rev 1998. 62: 130-180

[46]   Jones JM. Laboratory diagnosis of invasive candidiasis. Clin Microbiol Rev 1990. 3: 32-45.

[47]   Mille C, Janbon G, Delplace F, Ibata-Ombetta S, Gaillardin C, Strecker G, Jouault T, Trinel PA and Poulain D. Inactivation of CaMIT1 inhibits Candida albicans phospholipomannan beta-mannosylation, reduces virulence, and alters cell wall protein beta-mannosylation. J Biol Chem 2004. 279: 47952-47960.

[48]   Ruiz-Herrera J, Elorza MV, Valentin E and Sentandreu R, Molecular organization of the cell wall of Candida albicans and its relation to pathogenicity. FEMS Yeast Res 2006. 6: 14-29.

[49]   Tronchin G, Poulain D, Herbaut J and Biguet J. Localization of chitin in the cell wall of Candida albicans by means of wheat germ agglutinin. Fluorescence and ultrastructural studies. Eur J Cell Biol 1981. 26: 121-128.

[50]   Molano J, Bowers B and Cabib E. Distribution of chitin in the yeast cell wall. An ultrastructural and chemical study. J Cell Biol 1980. 85: 199-212.

[51]   Lopez-Ribot JL, Casanova M, Murgui A and Martinez JP. Antibody response to Candida albicans cell wall antigens. FEMS Immunol Med Microbiol 2004. 41: 187-196.

[52] Nicholls S, MacCallum DM, Kaffarnik FA, Selway L, Peck SC, Brown AJ. Activation of the heat shock transcription factor Hsf1 is essential for the full virulence of the fungal pathogen Candida albicans. Fungal Genet Biol. 2011; 48: 297-305.

[53] Berman J, Sudbery PE. Candida albicans: a molecular revolution built on lessons from budding yeast. Nat Rev Genet. 2002; 3: 918-30.

[54] Staib P, Morschhäuser J. Chlamydospore formation in Candida albicans and Candida dubliniensis an enigmatic developmental programme. Mycoses. 2007; 50: 1-12

[55] Soll DR. Why does *Candida albicans* switch? FEMS Yeast Res. 2009; 9: 973-89.

[56] Odds FC. Candida and Candidosis. second ed. Bailliere Tindall, London, United Kingdom, 1988.

[57] Sudbery PE. Growth of Candida albicans hyphae. Nat Rev Microbiol. 2011; 9 :

737-48. doi: 10. 1038/nrmicro2636.

[58] Albuquerque P, Casadevall A. Quorum sensing in fungi. A review Med Mycol. 2012; 50: 337-45.

[59] Jacobsen ID, Wilson D, Wächtler B, Brunke S, Naglik JR, Hube B. Candida albicans dimorphism as a therapeutic target. Expert Rev Anti Infect Ther. 2012; 10: 85-93.

[60] Saville SP, Lazzell AL, Monteagudo C, Lopez-Ribot JL. Engineered control of cell morphology in vivo reveals distinct roles for yeast and filamentous forms of *Candida albicans* during infection. Eukaryot Cell. 2003; 2: 1053-60.

[61] Garcia MC, Lee JT, Ramsook CB, Alsteens D, Dufrêne YF, Lipke PN. A role for amyloid in cell aggregation and biofilm formation. PLoS One. 2011; 6: e17632.

[62] Verstrepen KJ, Klis FM. Flocculation, adhesion and biofilm formation in yeasts. Mol Microbiol. 2006; 60: 5-15.

[63] Zordan R, Cormack B. Adhesins on Opportunistic Fungal Pathogens. In Candida and candisiasis, 2nd ed; Calderone RA, Clancy CJ. eds. ASM Press, Washington, DC, pp 243-259, 2012.

[64]   Murciano C, Moyes DL, Runglall M, Tobouti P, Islam A, Hoyer LL, et al. Evaluation of the role of Candida albicans agglutinin-like sequence (Als) proteins in human oral epithelial cell interactions. PLoS One. 2012; 7: e33362.

[65]   Staab JF, Bradway SD, Fidel PL, Sundstrom P. Adhesive and mammalian transglutaminase substrate properties of Candida albicans Hwp1. Science. 1999; 283: 1535-8.

[66]   Sundstrom P, Balish E, Allen CM. Essential role of the Candida albicans transglutaminase substrate, hyphal wall protein 1, in lethal oroesophageal candidiasis in immunodeficient mice. J Infect Dis. 2002; 185: 521-30.

[67]   Nobile CJ, Schneider HA, Nett JE, Sheppard DC, Filler SG, Andes DR, and al. Complementary adhesin function in C albicans biofilm formation. Curr Biol. 2008; 18: 1017-24.

[68]   Naglik JR, Moyes DL, Wächtler B, Hube B. Candida albicans interactions with epithelial cells and mucosal immunity. Microbes Infect. 2011; 13: 963-76.

[69]   Zhu W, Filler SG. Interactions of Candida albicans with epithelial cells. Cell Microbiol. 2010; 12: 273-82.

[70]   Zakikhany K, Naglik JR, Schmidt-Westhausen A, Holland G, Schaller M, Hube B. In vivo transcript profiling of *Candida albicans* identifies a gene essential for interepithelial dissemination. Cell Microbiol. 2007; 9: 2938-54.

[71]   Phan QT, Fratti RA, Prasadarao NV, Edwards JE Jr, Filler SG. N-cadherin mediates endocytosis of *Candida albicans* by endothelial cells. J Biol Chem. 2005; 280: 10455-61.

[72]   Park H, Myers CL, Sheppard DC, Phan QT, Sanchez AA, E Edwards J, et al. Role of the fungal Ras-protein kinase. A pathway in governing epithelial cell interactions during oropharyngeal candidiasis. Cell Microbiol. 2005; 7: 499-510.

[73]   Sun JN, Solis NV, Phan QT, Bajwa JS, Kashleva H, Thompson A and al. Host cell invasion and virulence mediated by Candida albicans Ssa1. PLoS Pathog. 2010; 6: e1001181

[74]   Wächtler B, Wilson D, Haedicke K, Dalle F, Hube B. From attachment to damage: defined genes of Candida albicans mediate adhesion, invasion and

damage during interaction with oral epithelial cells. PLoS One. 2011; 6: e17046.

[75] Fanning S, Mitchell AP. Fungal biofilms. PLoS Pathog. 2012; 8: e1002585.

[76] Finkel JS, Mitchell AP. Genetic control of Candida albicans biofilm development. Nat Rev Microbiol. 2011; 9: 109-18.

[77] Robbins N, Uppuluri P, Nett J, Rajendran R, Ramage G, Lopez-Ribot JL, et al. Hsp90 governs dispersion and drug resistance of fungal biofilms. PLoS Pathog. 2011; 7: e1002257

[78] Kumamoto CA. Molecular mechanisms of mechanosensing and their roles in fungal contact sensing. Nat Rev Microbiol. 2008; 6: 667-73.

[79] Brand A, Shanks S, Duncan VM, Yang M, Mackenzie K, Gow NA. Hyphal orientation of Candida albicans is regulated by a calcium-dependent mechanism. Curr Biol. 2007; 17: 347-52.

[80] Wächtler B, Citiulo F, Jablonowski N, Förster S, Dalle F, Schaller M, and al. Candida albicans-epithelial interactions: dissecting the roles of active penetration, induced endocytosis and host factors on the infection process. PLoS One. 2012; 7: e36952.

[81] Naglik JR, Challacombe SJ, Hube B. Candida albicans secreted aspartyl proteinases in virulence and pathogenesis. Microbiol Mol Biol Rev. 2003; 67: 400-28. doi: 10. 1128/MMBR. 67. 3. 400-428. 2003.

[82] Davis DA. How human pathogenic fungi sense and adapt to pH: the link to virulence. Curr Opin Microbiol. 2009; 12: 365-70.

[83] Mühlschlegel FA, Fonzi WA. PHR2 of Candida albicans encodes a functional homolog of the pH-regulated gene PHR1 with an inverted pattern of pH-dependent expression. Mol Cell Biol. 1997; 17: 5960-7.

[84] Vylkova S, Carman AJ, Danhof HA, Collette JR, Zhou H, Lorenz MC. The fungal pathogen Candida albicans autoinduces hyphal morphogenesis by raising extracellular pH. MBio. 2011; 2: e00055-11.

[85] Mayer FL, Wilson D, Jacobsen ID, Miramón P, Große K, Hube B. The novel Candida albicans transporter Dur31 is a multi-stage pathogenicity factor. PLoS Pathog. 2012; 8: e1002592.

[86]   Brock M. Fungal metabolism in host niches. Curr Opin Microbiol. 2009; 12: 371-6.

[87]   Frohner IE, Bourgeois C, Yatsyk K, Majer O, Kuchler K. Candida albicans cell surface superoxide dismutases degrade host-derived reactive oxygen species to escape innate immune surveillance. Mol Microbiol. 2009; 71: 240-52.

[88]   Lorenz MC, Bender JA, Fink GR. Transcriptional response of Candida albicans upon internalization by macrophages. Eukaryot Cell. 2004; 3: 1076-87

[89]   Ghosh S, Navarathna DH, Roberts DD, Cooper JT, Atkin AL, Petro TM, and al. Arginine-induced germ tube formation in Candida albicans is essential for escape from murine macrophage line RAW 264. 7. Infect Immun. 2009; 77: 1596-605

[90]   Pittet D, Monod M, Suter P, Frenk E, and Auckenthaler R. Candida colonization and subsequent infections in critically ill surgical patients. Ann Surg 1994; 220: 751-758.

[91]   Edwards JE, Bodey GP, Bowden RA, Buchner T, de Pauw BE, Filler SG, et al. International conference for the development of a consensus on the management and prevention of severe candidal infections. Clin Infect Dis 1997; 25: 43-59.

[92]   Vincent JL, Bihari DJ, Suter PM, et al. The prevalence of nosocomial infection in intensive care units in Europe. Results of the European Prevalence of Infection in Intensive Care (EPIC) Study. EPIC International Advisory Committee. JAMA 1995; 274: 639-44.

[93]   Wey SB, Motomi M, Pfaller MA, Woolson RF, Wenzel RP. Hospital acquired candidemia. The attributable mortality and excess length of stay. Arch Intern Med 1988; 148: 2642-5.

[94]   Eggimann P, Pittet D. Candidoses en réanimation Réanimation .2002 ; 11 : 209-21© 2002 Éditions scientifiques et médicales Elsevier SAS.

[95]   Solomkin JS, Flohr AB, Simmons RL. Indications for therapy for fungemia in postoperative patients. Arch Surg. 1982; 117: 1272-5.

[96]   Eggimann P, Francioli P, Bille J, Schneider R, Wu MM, Chapuis G; et al. Fluconazole prophylaxis prevents intra-abdominal candidiasis in high-risk surgical patients. Crit Care Med 1999; 27: 1066-72.

[97]   Rangel-Frausto MS, Wiblin T, Blumberg HM, Saiman L, Patterson J, Rinaldi M and al. National epidemiology of mycoses survey: variations in rates of bloodstream infections due to Candida species in seven surgical intensive care units and six neonatal intensive care units. Clin Infect Dis 1999; 29: 253-8.

[98]   Pittet D, Li N, Woolson RF, Wenzel RP. Microbiological factors influencing the outcome of nosocomial bloodstream infections. A six-year validated, population-based model. Clin Infect Dis 1997; 24: 1068-78.

[99]   Dubau B, Triboulet S, Winnock S. Practical use of the colonization index. Ann Fr Anesth Reanim 2001, 20: 418-420.

[100]   Garbino J, Lew PD, Romand JA, Hugonnet S, Auckenthaler R, Pittet D. Prevention of severe Candida infections in non-neutropenic, high-risk, critically ill patients. A randomized, double blind, placebo-controlled trial in SDD-treated patients. Intensive Care Med 2002, 28: 1708-1717.

[101]   Chabasse D. Interest of yeast counts in urine. Revue de la littérature et résultats préliminaires d'une enquête multicentrique réalisée dans 15 centers hospitaliers universitaires. Ann Fr Anesth Reanim 2001, 20: 400-406.

[102]   Charles PE, Dalle F, Aube H, Doise JM, Quenot JP, Aho LS and al. Candida spp colonization significance in critically ill medical patients: a prospective study. Intensive Care Med 2005, 31: 393-400

[103]   Normand S, Francois B, Darde ML, Bouteille B, Bonnivard M, Preux PM, and al.Oral nystatin prophylaxis of Candida spp. colonization in ventilated critically-ill patients. Intensive Care Med 2005, 31: 1466-1468.

[104]   Agvald-Ohman C , Klingspor L, Hjelmqvist H, Edlund C. Invasive candidiasis in long-term patients at a multidisciplinary intensive care unit: Candida colonization index, risk factors, treatment and outcome. Scand J Infect Dis. 2008; 40(2): 145-53.

[105]   Senn L, Eggimann P, Ksontini R, Pascual A, Demartines N, Bille J, and al. Caspofungin for prevention of intra-abdominal candidiasis in high-risk surgical patients. Intensive Care Med 2009, 35(5): 903-8.

[106]   Samonis G, Gikas A, Anaissie EJ, Vrenzos G, Maraki S, Tselentis Y, and al. Prospective evaluation of effects of broad-spectrum antibiotics on

gastrointestinal yeast colonization of humans. Antimicrob Agents Chemother 1993; 37: 51-3.

[107] Wey SB, Mori M, Pfaller MA, Woolson RF, Wenzel RP. Risk factors for hospital-acquired candidemia. A matched case- control study. Arch Intern Med 1989; 149: 2349-53.

[108] Fraser VJ, Jones M, Dunkel J, Storfer S, Medoff G, Dunagan WC. Candidemia in a tertiary care hospital: epidemiology, risk factors, and predictors of mortality. Clin Infect Dis 1992; 15: 414-21

[109] Talarmin J P, Boutoille D, Tattevin P, et al. Epidemiology of candidemia: a one-year prospective observational study in western France. Médecine Et Maladies Infectieuses 2009: 877-885.

[110] Pramayon S. Systemic candidiasis in intensive care: diagnostic and therapeutic difficulties, current consensus attitude. Sciences pharmaceutiques 2001 (Thesis).

[111] Blumberg HM, Jarvis WR, Soucie JM, Edwards JE, Patterson JE, Pfaller MA and al. Risk factors for candidal bloodstream infections in surgical intensive care unit patients: The NEMIS prospective multicenter study. The National Epidemiology of Mycosis Survey. Clinical Infectious Diseases. 2001; 33: 177-186

[112] Gauzit R. Epidemiology and risk factors of systemic candidiasis in the intensive care unit. Ann. Fr. Anesth. Réanim, 2001, 20: 394-399.

[113] Garber G. An overview of fungal infections. Drugs 2001, 61, Suppl. I: 1-12.

[114] Dupont H. Yeasts in intensive care. In: Sfar editor. Conférence d'actualisation. Congrès national d'anesthésie et de réanimation 2007; 415-32.

[115] Dupont H, Bourichon A, Paugam-Burtz C, et al. Can yeast isolation in peritoneal fluid be predicted in intensive care unit patients with peritonitis? Crit Care Med 2003; 31: 752-757.

[116] Lavigne J. P and Sotto A. Candiduria, Prog. Urol. 2005; 15: 213-216.

[117] Ang BSP, Telenti A, King B and al. Candidemia from a urinary tract source: microbiological aspects and clinical significance. Clin. Infect. Dis 1993; 17: 662-666.

[118] Kauffman CA, Vazquez JA, Sobel JD, et al. Prospective multicenter surveillance study of funguria in hospitalized patients. Clin. Infect. Dis 2000; 30 14-18.

[119] Sobel JD. Practice guidelines for the treatment of fungal infections. For the mycoses study group. Infectious diseases society of America. Clin. Infect. Dis. 2000; 30: 652.

[120] Laupland KB, Bagshaw SM, Gregson DB et al. Intensive care unit-acquired urinary tract infections in a regional critical care system. Crit. Care 2005; 9: R60-R65.

[121] Alvarez-Lerma F, Nolla-Sallas J, Leon C and al. Candiduria in critically ill patients admitted to intensive care medical units. Intensive Care Med. 2003; 29: 1069-1076.

[122] Nassoura Z, Ivatury RR, Simon RJ, et al. Candiduria as an early marker of disseminated infection in critically ill surgical patients: the role of fluconazole therapy. J. Trauma 1993; 35: 290-294.

[123] Soll DR. Candida commensalism and virulence: the evolution of phenotypic plasticity. Acta Trop. 2002; 2: 101-10.

[124] Calderone RA, Fonzi WA. Virulence factors of Candida albicans. Trends Microbiol 2001; 7: 327-35.

[125] Douglas LJ. Candida biofilms and their role in infection. Trends Microbiol 2003; 1: 30-6.

[126] Ramage G, Saville SP, Thomas DP, López-Ribot JL. Candida biofilms: an update. Eukaryot Cell 2005; 4: 633-8.

[127] Stéphan F, Bah MS, Desterke C, Rézaiguia-Delclaux S, Foulet F, Duvaldestin P and al. Molecular diversity and routes of colonization of Candida albicans in a surgical intensive care unit, as studied using microsatellite markers. Clin Infect Dis 2002; 12 : 1477-83

[128] Deorukhkar SC, Saini S, Mathew S. (2014). Non-albicans Candida Infection: An emerging threat. Interdisciplinary Perspectives on Infectious Diseases 2014(2014): 7.

[129] Netea MG, Marodi L. (2010). Innate immune mechanisms for recognition and uptake of Candida species. Trends Immunol 31(9): 346-353.

[130] Fidel Jr PL (2002). Immunity to Candida. Oral Dis 8(suppl 2): 69-75.

[131] Greenfield RA. (1992). Host defense system interaction with Candida. J Med Vet Mycol 30(2): 89-104.

[132] Enwonwu CO, Meeks VI (1996). Oral candidiasis HIV and saliva glucocorticoids. Am J Pathol 148(4): 1313-1338.

[133] De Repentigny L, Lewandowski D, Jolicoeur P. (2004). Immunopathogenesis of oropharyngeal candidiasis in human immunodeficiency virus infection. Clin Microbiol Rev 17(4): 729- 759.

[134] Edgerton M, Koshlukova SE, Lo TE, Chrzan BG, Straubinger RM, et al. (1998). Candidacidal activity of salivary histatins. Identification of a histatin 5-binding protein on Candida albicans. J Biol Chem 273(32): 20438-20447.

[135] Helmerhorst EJ, van't, Hof W, Breeuwer P, Veerman EC, Abee T, et al. (2001). Characterization of histatin 5 with respect to amphipathicity, hydrophobicity, and effects on cell and mitochondrial membrane integrity excludes a candidacidal mechanism of pore formation. J Biol Chem 276(8): 5643-5649.

[136] Van der Meer JW, van de Veerdonk FL, Joosten LA, Kullberg BJ, Netea MG (2010). Severe Candida spp. infections: new insights into natural immunity. Int J Antimicrob Agents 36(Suppl 2): S58-S62.

[137] Duggan S, Leonhardt I, Hünniger K, Kurzai O. (2015). Host response to Candida albicans bloodstream infection and sepsis. Virulence 6 (4): 316-326.

[138] Demirezen Ş, Dönmez HG, Özcan M, Beksaç MS (2015). Evaluation of the relationship between fungal infection, neutrophil leukocytes and macrophages in cervicovaginal smears: Light microscopic examination. J Cytol 32(2): 79-84.

[139] Naglik JR (2014). Candida Immunity. New J Sci 2014 (2014): 27.

[140] Ha JF, Italiano CM, Heath CH, Shih SS, Rea S, and al. (2011). Candidemia and invasive candidiasis: A review of the literature for the burns surgeon. Burns 37(2): 181-195.

[141] Netea MG, Gow NA, Munro CA, Bates S, Collins C, Ferwerda G, Hobson RP, Bertram G, Hughes HB, Jansen T, Jacobs L, Buurman ET, Gijzen K, Williams

DL, Torensma R, McKinnon A, MacCallum DM, Odds FC, Van der Meer JW, Brown AJ and Kullberg BJ .2006. Immune sensing of Candida albicans requires cooperative recognition of mannans and glucans by lectin and toll-like receptors. The Journal of clinical investigation. 116, 1642-1650.

[142] Poulain D, Jouault T. Candida albicans cell wall glycans, host receptors and responses: elements for decisive crosstalk. Current Opinion in Microbiology 2004 Aug;7(4):342-9.

[143] Coogan MM, Sweet SP, Challacombe SJ. Immunoglobulin A (IgA), IgA1, and IgA2 antibodies to Candida albicans in whole and parotid saliva in human immunodeficiency virus infection and AIDS. American Society for Microbiology Journals. Published online March 1, 1994.

[144] Astrid ML, Aniki R, Jack DS, Markus R, Peter GP , Claudio V, Haran TS, Iwona TO, John JH, Rex JK. Ocular Manifestations of Candidemia. Clinical Infectious Diseases, Volume 53, Issue 3, 1 August 2011, Pages 262-268.

[145] http: //assistancetaysir. Blogspot. com /2011/05/fond-doeil-en-cas dendophtalmie-levures. html

[146] Fisher JF, Chew WH, Shadomy S, Duma RJ, Mayhall LCG, House WC. Urinary tract infections due to Candida albicans. Rev. Infect. Dis, 1982, 4, 1107- 1116.

[147] Kozinn P J, Aschdjian STC, Golberg PK, WISE GJ, Toni EF, Seelig M. S. Advances in the diagnosis of renal candidiasis. J. Urol, 1978, 119, 184-187.

[148] Hurley R, Winner HI. Experimental renal moniliasis in the mouse. J. Pathol, 1963, 86, 75-82.

[149] Fisher JF, Mayhall CG, Duma RJ, Shadomy S, Shadomy J, Walligton C. Fungus ball of the urinary tract. South Med. J, 1979, 72, 1281-1284.

[150] Stening SG, Chritie WJ. "Fungus ball" of the urinary blad-der Med. J. Aust. 1972, 1, 372-373

[151] Humbert G, Brasseur P. Les candiduries : du diagnostic au traitement. Progrès en Urologie (1999), 9, 50- 56.

[152] Tomashefski JF, Abramowsky CR. Candida-associated renal papillary necrosis. Am. J. Clin. Pathol. 1981, 75, 190-194.

[153] http: //fn. bmj. com/content/89/4/F376. 4

[154] Badiee P, Amirghofran AA, Ghazi NM, Shafa M, Nemati MH. Incidence and outcome of documented fungal endocarditis. Int Cardiovasc Res J. 2014; 8(4): 152-155.

[155] Pierrotti LC, Baddour LM. Fungal endocarditis, 1995-2000. Chest. 2002; 122(1): 302-310

[156] Rubinstein E, Lang R. Fungal endocarditis. Eur Heart J. 1995; 16(Suppl B): 84-89.

[157] Seo GW, Seol SH, No TH, Jeong HJ, Kim TJ, Kim JK and al. Acute myocardial infarction caused by coronary embolism from Aspergillus endocarditis. Intern Med. 2014; 53(7): 713-716.

[158] Fernàndez Guerrero ML, Àlvarez B, Manzarbeitia F, Renedo G. Infective endocarditis at autopsy: a review of pathologic manifestations and clinical correlates. Medicine (Baltimore) 2012; 91(3): 152-164.

[159] Demir T, Ergenoglu MU, Ekinci A, Tanrikulu N, Sahin M, Demirsoy E. Aspergillus flavus endocarditis of the native mitral valve in a bone marrow transplant patient. Am J Case Rep. 2015; 16: 25-30.

[160] Ellis ME, Al-Abdely H, Sandridge A, Greer W, Ventura W. Fungal endocarditis: evidence in the world literature, 1965-1995. Clin Infect Dis. 2001; 32(1): 50-62.

[161] Toyoda S, Tajima E, Fukuda R, Masawa T, Inami S, Amano H and al. Early surgical intervention and optimal medical treatment for Candida parapsilosis endocarditis. Intern Med. 2015; 54(4): 411-413.

[162] Cornely OA, Bassetti M, Calandra T, Garbino J, Kullberg BJ, Lortholary O, and al. ESCMID Fungal Infection Study Group ESCMID* guideline for the diagnosis and management of Candida diseases 2012: non-neutropenic adult patients. Clin Microbiol Infect. 2012; 18(Suppl 7): 19-37.

[163] Rabinovici R, Szewczyk D, Ov Adia P, Greenspan JR, Siv Alingam JJ. Candida pericarditis: clinical profile and treatement. Ann. Thorac. Surg, 1997, 63: 1200-1204.

[164] Cornely OA, Gachot B, Akan H, Bassetti M, Uzun O, Kibbler C, et al. Epidemiology and outcome of fungemia in a cancer Cohort of the Infectious Diseases Group (IDG) of the European Organization for Research and

Treatment of Cancer (EORTC 65031). Clin Infect Dis Off Publ Infect Dis Soc Am. 2015 Aug 1; 61(3): 324-31.

[165] Pagano L, Mele L, Fianchi L, Melillo L, Martino B, D'Antonio D, and al. Chronic disseminated candidiasis in patients with hematologic malignancies. Clinical features and outcome of 29 episodes. Haematologica 2002; 87: 535-54

[166] De Pauw B, Walsh TJ, Donnelly JP, Stevens DA, Edwards JE, Calandra T, and al. Revised definitions of invasive fungal disease from the European Organization for Research and Treatment of Cancer/Invasive Fungal Infections Cooperative Group and the National Institute of Allergy and Infectious Diseases Mycoses Study Group (EORTC/MSG) Consensus Group. Clin Infect Dis 2008; 46: 1813-1821

[167] Metser U, Haider MA, Dill-Macky M, Atri M, Lockwood G, Minden M. Fungal liver infection in immunocompromised patients: depiction with multiphasic contrast-enhanced helical CT. Radiology 2005; 235: 97-105.

[168] Matuszkiewicz-Rowinska J. Update on fungal peritonitis and its treatment. Perit Dial Int 2009; 29 (Suppl. 2): S161-S165.

[169] Levallois J, Nadeau-Fredette AC, Labbé AC, and al. Ten-year experience with fungal peritonitis in peritoneal dialysis patients: antifungal susceptibility patterns in a North-American center. Int J Infect Dis 2012; 16: e41-e43.

[170] Miles R, Hawley CM, McDonald SP, et al. Predictors and outcomes of fungal peritonitis in peritoneal dialysis patients. Kidney Int 2009; 76: 622-628.

[171] Pappas PG, Kauffman CA, Andes D, et al. Clinical Practice Guidelines for the management of candidiasis: 2009 update by the Infectious Diseases Society of America. Clin Infect Dis 2009; 48: 503-535

[172] Lenz P, Conrad B, Kucharzik T, et al. Prevalence, associations, and trends of biliary-tract candidiasis: a prospective observational study. Gastrointest Endosc 2009; 70: 480-487.

[173] Diebel LN, Raafat AM, Dulchavsky SA, Brown WJ. Gallbladder and biliary tract candidiasis. Surgery 1996; 120: 760-764.

[174] Trikudanathan G, Navaneethan U, Vege SS. Intra-abdominal fungal infections complicating acute pancreatitis: a review. Am J Gastroenterol 2011; 106: 1188-1192.

[175] Vege SS, Gardner TB, Chari ST, et al. Outcomes of intra-abdominal fungal vs. bacterial infections in severe acute pancreatitis. Am J Gastroenterol 2009; 104: 2065-2070.

[176] Hoerauf A, Hammer S, Möller-Myhsok B, Rupprecht H. Intra-abdominal Candida infection during acute necrotizing pancreatitis has a high prevalence and is associated with increased mortality. Crit Care Med 1998; 26: 2010-2015.

[177] Fernandez-Sola J, Junque A, Estruch R, Monforte R, Torres A, Urbano-Marquez A. High alcohol intake and prognostic factor for community acquired pneumonia. Arch Intern Med 1995; 155: 1649-54.

[178] Wheat LJ. Infection and diabetes mellitus. Diabetes Care 1980; 3: 187-97.

[179] Mattiuzzi G, Giles FJ. Management of intracranial fungal infections in patients with haematological malignancies. Br J Haematol. 2005; 131(3): 287.

[180] Fennelly AM, Slenker AK, Murphy LC, Moussouttas M, DeSimone JA. Candida cerebral abscesses: a case report and review of the literature. Med Mycol. 2013 Oct; 51(7): 779-84.

[181] Sànchez-Portocarrero J, Pérez-Cecilia E, Corral O, Romero-Vivas J, Picazo JJ. The central nervous system and infection by Candida species. Diagn Microbiol Infect Dis. 2000; 37(3): 169.

[182] Fernandez M, Moylett EH, Noyola DE, Baker CJ. Candidal meningitis in neonates: a 10-year review. Clin Infect Dis. 2000; 31(2): 458.

[183] Kauffman CA, Marr KA, Thorner AR. Candida osteoarticular infections. UpToDate (2018).

[184] Pihet M, Marot M. Biological diagnosis of candidiasis. RFL- Revue Francophone des laboratoires. V 43, N 450-March 2013. pp47-61.

[185] Freydiere AM, Guinet R, Boiron P. Yeast identification in the clinical microbiology laboratory: phenotypical methods. Med Mycol 2001; 39(1): 9-33.

[186] Sendid B, Ducoroy P, Francois N, et al. Evaluation of MALDI-TOF mass spectrometry for the identification of medically-important yeasts in the clinical laboratories of Dijon and Lille hospitals. Med Mycol 2012.

[187] Jabra-Rizk MA, Brenner TM, Romagnoli M, et al. Evaluation of a reformulated CHROMagar Candida. J Clin Microbiol 2001; 39(5): 2015-6.

[188] https: //twitter. com/educatihealth/status/652556662268555264

[189] Rousselle P, Freydiere AM, Couillerot PJ, and al. Rapid identification of Candida albicans by using Albicans ID and fluoroplate agar plates. J Clin Microbiol 1994; 32(12): 3034-6.

[190] Fuller DD, Davis Jr TE, Denys GA, et al. Evaluation of BACTEC MYCO/F Lytic medium for recovery of mycobacteria, fungi and bacteria from blood. J Clin Microbiol 2001; 39(8): 2933-6.

[191] Mackenzie DW. Serum tube identification of Candida albicans. J Clin Pathol 1962; 15(6): 563-5.

[192] Beheshti F, Smith AG, Krause GW. Germ tube and chlamydospore formation by Candida albicans on a new medium. J Clin Microbiol 1975; 2(4): 345-8.

[193] https: //en. slideshare. net/riadhhammedi9/candidose-15910217

[194] http: //untori2.   crihan. fr/unspf/2010_Lille_Aliouat_Parasitologie/res/CHLAMY. JP

[195] Quindos G, San Millan R, Robert R, et al. Evaluation of bichrolatex albicans, a new method for rapid identification of Candida albicans. Journal of Clinical Microbiology, 01 May 1997, 35(5): 1263-1265

[196] Marot-Leblond A, Beucher B, David S, et al. Development and evaluation of a rapid latex agglutination test using a monoclonal antibody to identify Candida dubliniensis colonies. J Clin Microbiol 2006; 44(1): 138-42.

[197] Crist AE, Dietz TJ, Kampschroer K. Comparison of the MUREX C albicans, Albicans-Sure, and BactiCard Candida test kits with the germ tube test for presumptive identification of Candida albicans. J Clin Microbiol 1996; 34(10): 2616-8.

[198] Freydiere AM, Buchaille L, Guinet R and al. Evaluation of latex reagents for rapid identification of Candida albicans and Candida krusei colonies. J Clin Microbiol 1997; 35(4): 877-80.

[199] Freydiere AM, Robert R, Ploton C, and al. Rapid identification of Candida glabrata with a new commercial test, GLABRATA RTT. J Clin Microbiol 2003; 41(8): 3861-3.

[200] Aubertine CL, Rivera M, Rohan SM, et al. Comparative study of the new colorimetric VITEK 2 yeast identification card versus the older fluorometric card and of CHROMagar Candida as a source medium with the new card. J Clin Microbiol 2006; 44(1): 227-8.

[201] Paugam A, Baixench MT, Taieb F, Champagnac C, Dupouy-Camet J. Emergence of Candida parapsilosis candidemia at Cochin hospital. Characterization of isolates and search for risk factors. Pathologie Biologie Volume 59, n° 1 pages 44-47 (February 2011).

[202] Arendrup MC, Bergmann OJ, Larsson L, et al. Detection of candidaemia in patients with and without underlying haematological disease. Clin Microbiol Infect 2010; 16(7): 855-62.

[203] Sendid B, Caillot D, Baccouch-Humbert B, et al. Contribution of the Platelia Candida-specific antibody and antigen tests to early diagnosis of systemic Candida tropicalis infection in neutropenic adults. J Clin Microbiol 2003; 41(10): 4551-8.

[204] Alam FF, Mustafa AS, Khan ZU. Comparative evaluation of (1,3)-beta-D-glucan, mannan and anti-mannan antibodies, and Candida species-specific snPCR in patients with candidemia. BMC Infect Dis 2007; 7: 103.

[205] Loeffler J, Henke N, Hebart H, et al. Quantification of fungal DNA by using fluorescence resonance energy transfer and the light cycler system. J Clin Microbiol 2000; 38(2): 586-90.

[206] Marr KA, Carter RA, Crippa F, Wald A, Corey L. Epidemiology and outcome of mould infections in hematopoietic stem cell transplant recipients. Clin Infect Dis 2002; 34 (7): 909-17.

[207] Wingard JR, Leather H. A new era of anti-fungal therapy. Biol Blood Marrow Trans-plant 2004; 10 (2): 73-90.

[208] Lacroix C, Dubach M, Feuilhad M. Echinocandins: a new class of antifungal agents. Médecine et Maladies Infectieuses . Volume 33, Issue 4, 1 April 2003, pages 183-191.

[209] Perfect JR, Marr KA, Walsh TJ, et al. Voriconazole treatment for less common, emerging, or refractory fungal infections. Clin In-fect Dis 2003; 36 (9): 1122-31.

[210] Paugam A. News on posaconazole. Med Mal Infect 2007; 37 (2): 71-6.

[211] Albengres E, Le Louet H, Tillement JP. Systemic antifungal agents. Drug interactions of clinical significance. Drug Saf 1998; 18(2): 83-97

[212] Hochart S , Barrier F , Durand-Joly I , Horrent S , Decaudin B , Odou P. Les antifongiques systémiques : Partie 1 : éléments pharmaceutiques. Le Pharmacien Hospitalier . Volume 43, Issue 173, June 2008, Pages 103-109.

[213] Marty FM, Cosimi LA, and Baden L. 2004. Breakthrough zygomycosis after voriconazole treatment in recipients of hematopoietic stem-cell transplants. N. Engl. J. Med. 350: 950-952.

[214] Pfaller MA, Messer SA, Hollis RJ, et al. Variation in susceptibility of bloodstream isolates of Candida glabrata to fluconazole according to patient age and geographic location in the United States in 2001 to 2007. J Clin Microbiol 2009; 47(10): 3185-90.

[215] Fohrer C, Nivoix Y, Moulin JC, Marçais A and Herbrecht R. Contributions of lipid derivatives of amphotericin B in the management of fungal infections. Thérapie 2006 May-June; 61 (3): 235-242

[216] Pappas PG, Kauffman CA, Andes DR, Clancy CJ, Marr KA, Ostrosky-Zeichner L, Reboli AC, Schuster MG, et al. Clinical Practice Guideline for the Management of Candidiasis: 2016. Update by the Infectious Diseases Society of America. I S

[217] Petri MG, Konig J, Moecke HP, et al. Epidemiology of invasive mycosis in ICU patients: a prospective multicenter study in 435 non-neutropenic patients. Paul-Ehrlich Society for Chemotherapy, Divisions of Mycology and Pneumonia Research. Intensive Care Med. 1997; 23: 317-25.

[218] Ibanez-Nolla J, Nolla-Salas M, Leon MA and al. Early diagnosis of candidiasis in non-neutropenic critically ill patients. J Infect. 2004; 48: 181-92.

[219] Garnacho-Montero J, León C, Almirante B, and al. Recomendaciones terapéuticas para infecciones fúngicas en el paciente crítico no neutropénico.

Conferencia de consenso. Conclusiones. Med Intensiva. 2005; 3(Suppl 1): 43-52.

[220] Ostrosky-Zeichner L, Sable C, Sobel J, et al. Multicenter retrospective development and validation of a clinical prediction rule for nosocomial invasive candidiasis in the intensive care setting. Eur J Clin Microbiol Infect Dis. 2007; 26: 271-6.

[221] Leon C, Ruiz-Santana S, Saavedra P and, al. A bedside scoring system ("Candida score") for early antifungal treatment in nonneutropenic critically ill patients with Candida colonization. Crit Care Med. 2006; 34: 730-7.

[222] Piarroux R, Grenouillet F, Balvay P, et al. Assessment of preemptive treatment to prevent severe candidiasis in critically ill surgical patients. Crit Care Med. 2004; 32: 2443-9.

[223] Calandra T, Marchetti O. Antifungal prophylaxis for intensive care unit patients: let's fine tune it. Intensive Care Med. 2002; 28: 1698-700.

[224] Pelz RK, Hendrix CW, Swoboda SM et al. Double-blind placebo-controlled trial of fluconazole to prevent candidal infections in critically ill surgical patients. Ann Surg. 2001; 233: 542-8.

[225] Cruciani M, de Lalla F, Mengoli C. Prophylaxis of Candida infections in adult trauma and surgical intensive care patients: a systematic review and meta-analysis. Intensive Care Med. 2005; 31: 1479-87

[226] Shorr AF, Chung K, Jackson WL, et al. Fluconazole prophylaxis in critically ill surgical patients: a meta-analysis. Crit Care Med. 2005; 33: 1928-35.

[227] Playford EG, Webster AC, Sorrell TC, Craig JC. Antifungal agents for preventing fungal infec-tions in non-neutropenic critically ill and surgical patients: systematic review and meta-analysis of randomized clinical trials. J Antimicrob Chemother. 2006; 57(4): 628-38

[228] De Waele JJ, Vogelaers D, Blot S, et al. Fungal infections in patients with severe acute pancreatitis and the use of prophylactic therapy. Clin Infect Dis. 2003; 37: 208-13.

[229] Horn DL, Neofytos D, Anaissie E, Fishman J, Steinbach WJ, Olyaei AJ, Marr KA,2 Pfaller M, Chang CH, and Webster K. Epidemiology and Outcomes of

Candidemia in 2019 Patients: Data from the Prospective Antifungal Therapy Alliance Registry Clinical Infectious Diseases 2009; 48: 1695-703.

[230] Bassetti M, Merelli M, Righi E, Diaz-Martin A, Rosello A M, Luzzati R, Parra A, Trecarichi E M, Sanguinetti M, Posteraro B, Garnacho-Montero J, Sartor A, Rello J, Tumbarellof M. Epidemiology, Species Distribution, Antifungal Susceptibility, and Outcome of Candidemia across Five Sites in Italy and Spain Journal of Clinical Microbiology p. 4167-4172 December 2013.

[231] Khelfaoui L, Djebellah N. Invasive candidiasis in the intensive care setting CHU Dr Benbadis de Constantine (January 2015December 2016). (Thesis).

[232] Gupta Priyanka, Prateek Shashank, Chatterjee1 Biswaroop, Kotwall Arti, Singh Amit K and Mittall Garima. Prevalence of Candidemia in ICU in a Tertiary Care Hospital in North India Int. J. Curr. Microbiol. App. Sci (2015) 4(6): 566-575.

[233] Arrache D, Madani K, Zait H, Achir I, Younsi N, Zebdi A, Bouahri L, Chaouche F, Hamrioui B. Fungemias diagnosed at the parasitology-mycology laboratory of CHU Mustapha d'Alger, Algeria (2004-2014). Journal de Mycologie Médicale. Volume 25, Issue 3, September 2015, Pages 237-238.

[234] Tessier X. Epidemiology of candidemias at Bordeaux University Hospital from April 30, 2012 to March 30, 2016. Human medicine and pathology. 2017.

[235] Sasso M, Roger C, Sasso M, Poujol H, Barbar S, Lefrant J-Y and al. Changes in the distribution of colonizing and infecting Candida spp. isolates, antifungal drug consumption and susceptibility in a French intensive care unit: A 10-year study. Mycoses. 2017 Jul 31.

[236] Tadec L, Talarmin J-P, Gastinne T, Bretonnière C, Miegeville M, Le Pape P, and al. Epidemiology, risk factor, species distribution, antifungal resistance and outcome of Candidemia at a single French hospital: a 7-year study. Mycoses. 2016 May; 59(5): 296-303.

[237] Nolla-Salas J, Sitges-Serra A, León-Gil C, Martínez-Gonzàlez J, León-Regidor MA, Ibàñez-Lucía P, Torres-Rodríguez JM. Candidemia in non-neutropenic critically ill patients: analysis of prognostic factors and assessment of systemic antifungal therapy. Study Group of Fungal Infection in the ICU. Intensive Care Med. 1997 Jan; 23(1): 23-30.

[238] Charles PE, Doise JM, Quenot JP. Medical and surgical patients' difference of outcome between candidemia in critically ill patients. Intensive care med 2003; 29: 2162-9.

[239] Colombo AL, Nucci M, Park BJ and al. Brazilian Network Candidemia Study Epidemiology of candidemia in Brazil: a nationwide sentinel surveillance of candidemia in eleven medical centers. J Clin Microbiol. 2006; 44(8): 2816-2823.

[240] Horn DL, Fishman JA, Steinbach WJ, Anaissie EJ, Marr KA, Olyaei AJ, and al. Presentation of the PATH Alliance® registry for prospective data collection and analysis of the epidemiology, therapy, and outcomes of invasive fungal infections. Diagn Microbiol. Infect Dis. 2007; 59: 407-14.

[241] Bitar D, Lortholary O, Dromer F, CoignardB, Che D. Invasive mycoses in metropolitan France, PMSI 2001-2010: incidence, case-fatality and trends. Bulletin Epidémiologique Hebdomadaire, 2013, n°. 12-13, p. 109-14

[242] Leroy O, Gangneux JP, Montravers P, and al. AmarCand Study Group Epidemiology, management, and risk factors for death of invasive Candida infections in critical care: a multicenter, prospective, observational study in France (2005-2006). Crit Care Med. 2009; 37(5): 1612-1618.

[243] Calandra T, Bille J, Schneider R, Mosimann F, Francioli P. Clinical significance of candida isolated from peritoneum in surgical patients. The Lancet 1989; 2: 1437-40.

[244] Montravers P, Gauzit R, Muller C, Marmuse JP, Fichelle A, Desmonts JM. Emergence of antibiotic-resistant bacteria in cases of peritonitis after intraabdominal surgery affects the efficacy of empirical antimicrobial therapy. Clin Infect Dis 1996; 23: 486-94.

[245] Sandven P, Bevanger L, Digranes A, Haukland HH, Mannsåker T, Gaustad P. Norwegian Yeast Study Group Candidemia in Norway (1991 to 2003): results from a nationwide study. J Clin Microbiol. 2006; 44(6): 1977-1981.

[246] Delestre G. Retrospective study of cases of candidal peritonitis developed in the surgical intensive care unit of Rouen University Hospital over a six-year period (2006-2011). Thesis 2013.

[247] Pappas PG. Invasive candidiasis. Infect Dis Clin North Am. 2006; 20(3): 485-506.

[248] Bouza E, Muñoz P. Epidemiology of candidemia in intensive care units. Int J Antimicrob Agents. 2008; 32(Suppl 2): S87-S91.

[249] Playford GE, Marriott D, Nguyen Q, et al. Candidemia in nonneutropenic critically ill patients: Risk factors for non-albicans Candida spp. Crit Care Med. 2008 Jul; 36(7) : 2034-9.

[250] Murray CK, Loo FL, Hospenthal DR, Cancio LC. Incidence of systemic fungal infection and related mortality following severe burns. Burns. December 2008; 34: 1108-1112.

[251] Zaoutis TE, Argon J, Chu J, Berlin JA, Walsh TJ, Feudtner C. The Epidemiology and Attributable Outcomes of Candidemia in Adults and Children Hospitalized in the United States: A Propensity Analysis. Clin Infect Dis. 2005; 41: 1232-9.

[252] Dylewksi ML, Baker M, Prelack K, Weber JM. The safety and efficacy of parenteral nutrition among pediatric patients with burn injuries. Pediatr Crit Care Med. 2013; 14: E120-E125.

[253] Mosier MJ, Pham TN, Klein MB, Gibran NS. Early enteral nutrition in burns: compliance with guidelines and associated outcomes in a multicenter study. J Burn Care Res. 2011; 32: 104-109

[254] Ben-Ami R, Weinberger M, Orni-Wasserlauff R, Schwartz D, Itzhaki A, Lazarovitch T, et al. Time to blood culture positivity as a marker for catheter-related candidemia. Journal of Clinical Microbiology. 2008; 46: 2222-2226.

[255] Tortorano AM, Kibbler C, Peman J, Bernhardt H, Klingspor L, Grillot R. Candidemia in Europe: epidemiology and resistance. Int J Antimicrob Agents. 2006; 27(5): 359-366. 639-644.

[256] Chow JK, Golan Y, Ruthazer R, Karchmer AW, Carmeli Y, Lichtenberg DA, et al. Risk factors for albicans and non-albicans candidemia in the intensive care unit. Critical Care Medicine. 2008; 36: 1993-1998.

[257] Ortiz Ruiz G, Osorio J, Valderrama S, Alvarez D, Elias Diaz R, Calderon J, et al. Risk factors for candidemia in nonneutropenic critical patients in Colombia. Medicina Intensiva. 2016; 40: 139-144

[258] Montagna MT, Caggiano G, Lovero G et al. Epidemiology of invasive fungal infections in the intensive care unit: Results of a multicenter Italian survey (AURORA Project) Infection. 2013; 41(3): 645-653.

[259] Yapar N, Pullukcu H, Avkan-Oguz V, et al. Evaluation of species distribution and risk factors of candidemia: a multicenter case-control study. Med Mycol. 2011; 49(1): 26-31.

[260] Gudlaugsson O, Gillespie S, Lee K, Berg JV, Hu J, Messer S, and al. Attributable Mortality of Nosocomial Candidemia, Revisited. Clin Infect Dis. 2003; 37: 1172-7.

[261] Pappas PG, Rex JH, Lee J, Hamill RJ, Larsen RA, Powderly W, et al. A Prospective Observational Study of Candidemia: Epidemiology, Therapy, and Influences on Mortality in Hospitalized Adult and Pediatric Patients. Clin Infect Dis. 2003; 37: 634-43.

[262] Ng KP , Saw TL, Na SL, Soo-Hoo TS. Systemic Candida infection in University hospital 1997-1999: The distribution of Candida biotypes and antifungal susceptibility patterns. Mycopathologia. 2001; 149(3): 141-6.

[263] Medrano DJ , Brilhante RS, Cordeiro Rde A, Rocha MF, Rabenhorst SH, Sidrim JJ. Candidemia in a Brazilian hospital: the importance of Candida parapsilosis. Rev Inst Med Trop Sao Paulo. 2006 Jan-Feb; 48(1): 17-20.

[264] Martino, P. C. Girmenia, A. Micozzi, R. Raccah, G. Gentile, M. Venditti, and F. Mandelli. 1993. Fungemia in patients with leukemia. Am. J. Med. Sci. 306: 225-232.

[265] Fridkin SK, Jarvis WR. Epidemiology of nosocomial fungal infections. Clin Microbiol Rev. 1996; 9: 499-511.

[266] Pfaller MA. Nosocomial Candidiasis: Emerging Species, Reservoirs, and Modes of Transmission. Clin Infect Dis. 1996; 22: S89-S94.

[267] Torres HA, Kontoyiannis DP, and Rolston KVI. 2004. High-dose fluconazole therapy for cancer patients with solid tumors and candidemia: an observational, noncomparative retrospective study. Support Care Cancer 12: 511-516

[268] Wingard, J. R. 1995. Importance of Candida species other than *C. albicans* as pathogens in oncology patients. Clin. Infect. Dis. 20: 115-125.

[269] Hoarau G, Picot S, Lemant J. Peytral J, Poubeau P, Zunic P, Mohr C, Coueffe X, Gerardin P, Antok E. Candidemia in intensive care unit, a 12 years' retrospective cohort study in reunion Island. Medecine et maladie infectieuse 48 - (2018) 414-418.

[270] Kreusch A, Karstaedt AS. Candidemia among adults in Soweto, South Africa, 1990-2007. Int J Infect Dis. 2013; 17(8): e621-e623.

[271] Poikonen E, Lyytikäinen O, Anttila VJ, Koivula I, Lumio J, Kotilainen P, Syrjälä H, Ruutu P. Secular trend in candidemia and the use of fluconazole in Finland, 2004-2007. BMC Infect Dis. 2010 Oct 28; 10: 312.

[272] Reboli AC, Rotstein C, Pappas PG, Chapman SW, Kett DH, Kumar D, and al. Anidulafungin versus Fluconazole for Invasive Candidiasis. N Engl J Med. 2007; 356: 2472-82.

[273] Andes DR, Safdar N, Baddley JW, Playford G, Reboli AC, Rex JH, et al. Impact of Treatment Strategy on Outcomes in Patients with Candidemia and Other Forms of Invasive Candidiasis: A Patient-Level Quantitative Review of Randomized Trials. Clin Infect Dis. 2012

[274] Colombo AL, Guimarães T, Sukienik T, Pasqualotto AC, Andreotti R, Queiroz-Telles F, et al. Prognostic factors and historical trends in the epidemiology of candidemia in critically ill patients: an analysis of five multicenter studies sequentially conducted over a 9-year period. Intensive Care Med. 2014; 40: 1489-98.

[275] Beraud G, Sendid B, Leroy-Coteau A, Faure K, Guery B. Registre des Candidémies au CHRU de Lille : Résultats à 1 an et adéquation de la prise en charge aux recommandations. Médecine et maladies infectieuses 39 (2009) S30.

[276] Rex JH,, Walsh TJ, Sobel JD, Filler SG, Pappas PG, Dismukes WE, Edwards JE. Practice guidelines for the treatment of candidiasis. Infectious Diseases Society of America. Clin Infect Dis. 2000 Apr; 30(4): 662-78.

[277] Arias S, Denis O, Montesinos I, Cherifi S, Miendje Deyi VY, Zech F. Epidemiology and mortality of candidemia both related and unrelated to the central venous catheter: A retrospective cohort study. European Journal of Clinical Microbiology & Infectious Diseases. 2017; 36: 501-507.

[278] Garnacho-Montero J, Diaz-Martin A, Garcia-Cabrera E, Ruiz Perez de Pipaon M, Hernandez-Caballero C, Lepe-Jimenez JA. Impact on hospital mortality of catheter removal and adequate antifungal therapy in Candida spp. bloodstream infections. The Journal of Antimicrobial Chemotherapy. 2013.

[279] Sendid B, Tabouret M, Poirot JL, and al. New enzyme immu-noassays for sensitive detection of circulating Candida albicans mannan and antimannan antibodies. J Clin Microbiol.1999;37:1510-7.

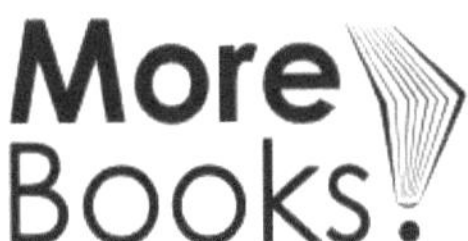

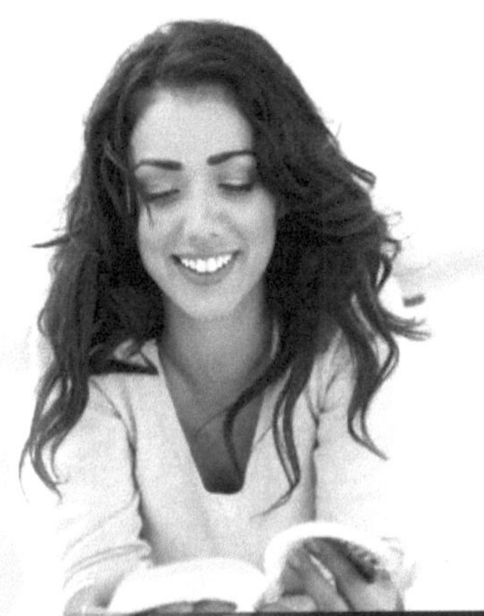

I want morebooks!

Buy your books fast and straightforward online - at one of world's fastest growing online book stores! Environmentally sound due to Print-on-Demand technologies.

Buy your books online at
www.morebooks.shop

Kaufen Sie Ihre Bücher schnell und unkompliziert online – auf einer der am schnellsten wachsenden Buchhandelsplattformen weltweit! Dank Print-On-Demand umwelt- und ressourcenschonend produziert.

Bücher schneller online kaufen
www.morebooks.shop

info@omniscriptum.com
www.omniscriptum.com

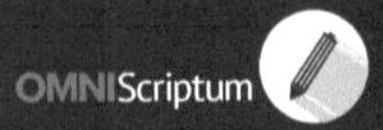

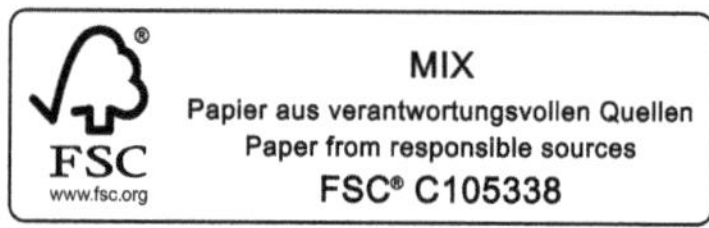

Printed by Books on Demand GmbH, Norderstedt / Germany